Emerginy
Therapies

Using Herbs and Nutraceutical Supplements for Small Animals

This AAHA publication has been brought to you through an educational grant from Merial Limited.

Emerging Therapies

Using Herbs and Nutraceutical Supplements for Small Animals

Susan G. Wynn, DVM

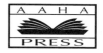

AAHA Press
12575 W. Bayaud Avenue
Lakewood, Colorado 80228

© 1999 by AAHA Press

ISBN 1-58326-010-2

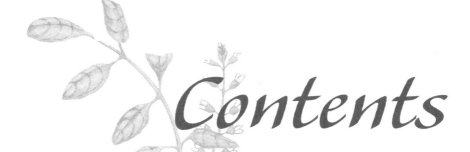

Contents

Tables

Figures

Foreword

We are entering an exciting era as we begin a new millennium, an era rich with opportunities for our patients, clients, and profession. Veterinary practitioners have opened their hearts, eyes, and minds to amazing new approaches to diagnose, treat, and heal the animals in our care. By recognizing and celebrating the wonderful bond between pets and people, veterinarians continually find new purpose for seeking out effective treatments regardless whether they are "high tech" or "high touch." In fact, more and more veterinarians are merging powerful new technological tools such as gene therapy, molecular modulators of immunity, cloning, laser surgery, and linear accelerator radiation therapy with healing modalities such as acupuncture and herbal and nutritional therapies that have been successfully used for generations.

To practice responsibly, veterinarians need up-to-date, valid information about alternative as well as technical treatment options. Fortunately, the American Animal Hospital Association and Dr. Susan Wynn have taken a bold, responsible, confident step to bring small animal practice into the twenty-first century with this balanced, informative book on botanic and nutraceutical therapies. Dr. Wynn penned this valuable book for the practitioner by recognizing and addressing known strengths and weaknesses of these complementary modalities. No other single author today has the background and the critical eye to provide such an honest assessment of these complementary and integrative therapies. In doing so, she has given us a wonderful resource to care for our patients not only from the mind, but also from the heart.

Practitioners in the new millennium will benefit immensely from this book for many reasons. First, more and more of our clients are using complementary therapies for their pets and for themselves. Approximately 4 billion people—80 percent of the world population—use herbal and botanical medicine, and many of these people seek this type of care for their pets. Conservative estimates indicate that one-third of all Americans routinely use alternative and complementary therapies, especially as a supplement to conventional health care methods. In fact, Americans visit alternative practitioners more often than physicians at a cost of more than $14 billion per year. In addition, Americans spend an additional $4 billion annually on alternative products such as vitamins and herbs.

This same trend is occurring in veterinary health care. Anyone who has practiced during the past five years can appreciate our clients' growing demand for herbal and botanical therapies. This is true especially in the treatment of cancer patients for whom traditional treatment options are limited and often toxic. Because these treatment modalities have been entrenched in traditional veterinary medicine as the standard of care, until recently there have been few Western-style studies to document the efficacy of nutraceutical and botanical treatments. However, this has changed in the past several years, as scientists have undertaken and published studies using traditional research methods to discover the efficacy of such treatments. With the results of each new study, our comfort level in using these treatments grows.

The number of herbs and other plant-based materials that can be used therapeutically is staggering. For example, results of a 25-year study (published in 1981) conducted by the US Department of Agriculture in conjunction with the National Cancer Institute focused on plants with anticancer properties. The study included 365 medicinal species and identified more than 1,000 pharmacologically active phytochemicals. Despite worldwide use of herbal and botanical treatments and research such as this, acceptance of these practices varies. Failure to at least recognize the potential benefit of botanical therapies is myopic for our profession and it stands in the way of many great opportunities for our patients.

This book not only discusses herbals and botanical therapies; it also reviews select aspects of nutritional therapy. The use of nutraceuticals revolves around the notion that nutrients prevent, support, and treat people and animals with cancer and a wide variety of other diseases. Indeed, nutrients have been used as a therapeutic tool for as long as records have been kept. A large quantity of data exists documenting the beneficial and adverse effects of nutrients, especially in veterinary medicine. Improving the diet of all animals has many beneficial consequences. Similarly, veterinarians' use of specific nutrients as a therapeutic tool is becoming more prominent.

The American Animal Hospital Association and Dr. Susan Wynn should be applauded by the entire profession for taking a responsible, scholarly step into the new millennium with this book and its invaluable benefit to people with pets, our patients, and an entire profession. I look forward to using this book in my practice as I search for new and better ways to provide compassionate care for pets and people in my celebration of the human–animal bond, which is the essence of our profession.

Gregory K. Ogilvie, DVM
Diplomate ACVIM (Specialties of Internal Medicine, Oncology)
Professor and Head of Medical Oncology
Department of Clinical Sciences
College of Veterinary Medicine and Biomedical Sciences
Colorado State University
Ft. Collins, Colorado

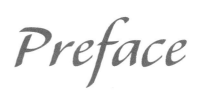

Preface

*R*emember the kid's game, Operation? The doctor is the quintessential mechanic, and the model is essentially that of modern medical practice.

Medical training often leads us to believe that parts can be medically or surgically removed, added, replaced, suppressed, or fixed in order to repair the failing system. There is only partial understanding of another model—one in which the doctor supports, tonifies, adjusts, balances, and waits—in order to fortify the sturdy adaptive responses already in use by a remarkable biological machine, the body.

We learn this model in veterinary school but soon forget in our clients' clamor for quick cures. Farmers and gardeners have understood this model throughout the ages. Nurturing a lush and well-producing plant isn't done simply by providing water and killing the bugs. Producers must read their individual fields and work out supplement plans appropriate to their crops, soil history, and time of year. Is it a stretch to manage individual dogs and cats in the same way? Isn't this what every veterinarian should do to keep pets healthy?

Truly holistic management involves close attention to environmental toxins (pesticide use, for instance) and immune or organ support and is still not the norm in clinical practice. Many veterinarians practice holistically, that is, treating the entire patient and not just the presenting disease.

However, veterinarians who practice truly complementary, holistic, or alternative medicine hold a more global view of the patient. Their work-ups often define such arcane concepts and unusual variables as season, time of day, total chemical load, miasm, food preferences, and body type, and treatments may involve "temperature" balancing or immune support.

If we remove things, fix things, replace things, and turn off symptoms, what are we doing to help the body adjust, balance, heal, and make use of our repairs? If we view the body as a machine, where is the fuel coming from? Supportive therapies, such as therapeutic nutrition, low-level toxin elimination, tonifying herbs, chiropractic, and acupuncture, supply a way to produce sustained responses and more lasting good health.

Our goal in medical treatment is a holistic—wholistic—one. Fixing one thing can decompensate another. We strive to avoid tunnel vision and use comprehensive medicine.

Many veterinarians are looking for new treatments that work from among that vast assortment of therapies labeled "alternative medicine." Many of these treatment systems require intense training—financial and time commitments many cannot make without seeing the promise in the modalities first. Acupuncture, chiropractic, homeopathy, and traditional Chinese medicine are among these therapies. I won't discuss them. This book will concentrate on therapies easily integrated into a standard conventional practice—nutraceuticals and herbs.

Although information on the popularity of alternatives, legal issues, and incorporation into conventional practice is introduced here, the meat of this text is more practical. The nutraceutical and botanical materia medica (chapters 4 and 5) offer indications, cautions, and dosages for the first time in the veterinary literature in this form. I hope that this book will help interested veterinary practitioners use certain alternative therapies—nutraceuticals and herbs—with a better understanding of the whole animal, using less toxic drugs that have more satisfactory long-term results than they have ever had before. Such therapies may change the face of small animal practice—they certainly changed mine.

Susan G. Wynn

Acknowledgments

A million thanks to all who helped with this book. Mary Kay, you know it wouldn't have happened without your inspiration. I had very supportive critics, as well—Chris Cowell, Helen Berschneider, Dave McCluggage, Nancy Scanlan, Darren Hawks, and Rob Silver—you guys whipped this project into tip-top shape. Also, to Jory Olsen—thanks for keeping me honest. And, to my friends and family, thanks for tolerating this, as well as my other eccentricities. And last, but certainly not least, I thank the indomitable Phylis Austin, who never tires of helping!

Chapter 1

Introduction

First, the patient, second the patient, third the patient, fourth the patient, fifth the patient, and then maybe comes the science.
—Bela Schick

Absence of evidence is not the same as evidence of absence.
—Linda Gooding, PhD.

Why Learn Therapies Not Yet Scientifically Proven?

Most practitioners experience the frustration of managing a refractory disease in a patient who deserves relief. Most would prefer to use medications or interventions that are 100% proven to work—and have no side effects. The real world of veterinary practice rarely gives such perfect solutions. Alternative—or unproven—diagnostic and treatment options expand our choices in managing chronic disease.

Alternative medicine has been described as "those interventions not taught widely at U.S. medical schools or generally available in U.S. hospitals" (Eisenberg et al. 1993). A recent editorial stated that there cannot be two kinds of medicine—conventional and alternative. Instead, "there is only medicine that has been adequately tested and medicine that has not, medicine that works and medicine that may or may not work" (Angell and Kassirer 1998). There is much to be said for this picture of medical care.

This book is not intended to promote unproven methods of care for animal patients with conditions successfully treated using proven methods. This book introduces new or unproven therapies for animals with chronic problems, animals who suffer severe side effects from conventional therapies, and animals who haven't been helped with standard veterinary medicine and whose owners may have run out of options. Chronic disease is, by definition, a failure of conventional methods.

The most practical reason for learning and using these unproven nutritional and herbal therapies assumes that potentially unique actions, and perhaps unique mechanisms, provide novel treatment strategies, effectively increasing our options. For instance, little in our current medical arsenal provides hepatoprotection and supports hepatic regeneration for liver insults of various types, yet milk thistle *(Silybum marianum)* has such effects and is quite nontoxic.

Yet another attraction of natural therapies may be perceived safety. Although herbs and nutritional supplements are not necessarily inherently safe, their history is marked with a notable lack of serious or sustained adverse effects, in contrast to popular pharmaceuticals. In the United States alone, recent reports estimate that 1.5 million people are hospitalized and up to 100,000 people die each year due to adverse drug effects (Moore, Psaty, and Furberg 1998). Doctors are not required to report adverse effects and neither are veterinarians; it is difficult to accurately estimate the problem, especially in veterinary medicine.

On the other hand, adverse effects of "natural" supplement use have been reported recently in the literature, possibly because of their increasing popularity. Again, doctors are not required to report dietary supplement toxicity, so the extent of these poisonings is simply not known. The World Health Organization (WHO) lists 8,985 adverse reactions from herbal preparations. Particularly difficult to discern are long-term causal relationships, such as cancer caused by long-term ingestion of a supplement. In the United Kingdom, 5,608 inquiries from 1991 to 1995 involved natural products; 77% of those involved asymptomatic cases, and about 80% of those involved vitamin/mineral-type supplements (Adverse Effects 1998).

A problem unique to herbal use is that patients and pet owners view natural medicine as do-it-yourself medicine and may be using supplements improperly—or dangerously. In three published reports on comfrey

(Symphytum officinale) toxicity, patients experienced veno-occlusive liver disease secondary to chronic ingestion of potentially high doses of the herb for 4 months to up to 3 years. Perhaps an additional inducement for veterinary practitioners to become well versed in herbal medicine is to prevent such lay-prescribed tragedies. Professionals trained in these areas are less likely to subscribe to the "if it's natural, it's safe" philosophy.

Still, herbs have been in use for thousands of years, with a supporting written tradition in some cultures. One herbalist stated that the death of a shaman (representing an oral tradition) is like the destruction of a library—in some cases a permanent loss unless ethnobotanical medicine can preserve the knowledge from isolated cultures. Whatever the fate of this body of knowledge, many herbs have effectively undergone mass efficacy and safety trials—similar to phase IV clinical trials of the Food and Drug Administration (FDA)—for quite a long time. Our job is to test this knowledge and apply it judiciously in animals until science catches up.

Putting Paradigms to Work

Although practitioners using herbs may refer to many existing studies describing active constituents as well as pharmacologic indications and interactions, herbs are an ancient and important component of most traditional medical cultures. Some well-documented cultural systems (Chinese and Ayurvedic) are thousands of years old; such long-standing traditions offer proven (in the cultural sense) diagnostic and treatment systems, which, though unfamiliar to Western practitioners, remain useful for patient care. Although these traditional paradigms may never be scientifically validated, they provide potentially useful guidance in the art of medicine.

Chinese medicine, for instance, uses Five Element and Eight Principle Theory, instructing that diseases and treatments may have characteristic imbalances relating to Wood, Fire, Earth, Metal, and Water, or Cold, Hot, Yin, Yang, Deficiency, Excess, Interior, and Exterior. Whether or not these concepts ever find scientific validity, they may be useful in prescribing for patients who have run the gamut of "scientifically proven" therapies. These systematic prescriptions may be learned only after intense training and practice, but they give the interested practitioner (and certainly the patient) yet more options for treatment.

Laying the Groundwork

Although we focus primarily on nutraceutical and herbal treatments in this book, the following definitions are provided for the sake of discussion. Every veterinarian should know the difference between *holistic* and *homeopathic*, for instance. Without a passing knowledge of the different therapies, we can be of no help to curious clients.

Defining Alternative Medicine

I define veterinary holistic medicine as follows:

Holistic veterinary medicine

The use of the least toxic intervention required to treat and balance a patient within the context of its historical and environmental situation, all in addition to the presenting complaint.

This definition describes what practitioners of natural and alternative therapies seek to accomplish; however, the concept does not necessarily involve the use of unconventional, emerging, or alternative therapies. In fact, most thoughtful veterinarians already practice holistic medicine.

Other related terms have been used over the years. The following are definitions from the *New Shorter Oxford English Dictionary* (Brown 1993):

alternative: "Stating or offering either of two things; expressing alternation, disjunctive. Of two things, mutually exclusive. Of one or more things, available in place of another. Designating a mode of life, system of knowledge and practice, organization, etc. purporting to represent a preferable and cogent alternative to that of the established social order."

integrative: Tending to "make entire or complete; make up, compose, constitute (a whole). Complete or perfect by addition of necessary parts. Put or bring together (parts) to form a whole; combine into a whole."

complementary: "Forming a complement, completing (of two or more things), complementing each other. Designating or pertaining to medicine that involves methods or means not recognized by the majority of medical practitioners, not given full official recognition, or not based on modern scientific knowledge."

unconventional: "Not limited or bound by convention or custom, diverging from accepted standards or models, unusual, unorthodox."

allopathic: "The treatment of disease by inducing an opposite condition (i.e., in the usual way). Opposite of homeopathy."

Readers are encouraged to find wording comfortable for them as they incorporate these new therapies into practice. For example, the proper use of the term "alternative" comes with no presumption about proof or lack thereof, or of attachment to therapeutic type. In May 1999, *Veterinary Economics* carried a news item titled "Veterinarians find alternative cancer treatments for cats and dogs"—this article referred to radioactive nasal implants. This is hardly related to the "natural" treatments usually considered part of "alternative medicine."

The strengths and limitations of each name should be clear. I prefer to apply none of these terms, using only the name of the modality being offered— there are only proven and unproven therapies, and the art of medicine often demands that we, as doctors, use any therapy appropriate for the patient.

Defining Individual Modalities

Individual modalities, such as homeopathy, naturopathy, and flower remedy therapy, are more restrictive types of treatment. The following is a short list of more common alternative modalities.

acupuncture: a method of stimulating certain points on the body by inserting needles to modulate physiologic functions in the prevention or treatment of disease. The American Veterinary Medical Association (AVMA) defines acupressure and acutherapy as "the examination and stimulation of specific points on the body of nonhuman animals by use of acupuncture needles, moxibustion, injections, low-level lasers, magnets, and a variety of other techniques for the diagnosis and treatment of numerous conditions in animals" (AVMA 1998).

aromatherapy: a branch of herbal medicine that uses "essential" oils of plants (obtained through steam distillation, cold pressing, or solvent extraction) to treat a variety of conditions. In human medicine, these oils are applied topically or by diffusion into room air.

Ayurvedic medicine: a traditional medical system of diagnosis and treatment originating in India thousands of years ago. Ayurveda uses a combination of diet, physical therapies, and indigenous herbs within a holistic approach.

chiropractic: "the examination, diagnosis, and treatment of nonhuman animals through manipulation and adjustments of specific joints and cranial sutures" (AVMA 1998).

detoxification: treatments designed to assist in an animal's recovery from toxic insults by increasing elimination of stored or ingested toxins through the liver, kidneys, GI tract, skin, or respiratory tract; also, a term that describes the side effects that may occur during this process.

flower remedies: originally called Bach flower remedies, these are specially prepared, very dilute extracts of certain flowers, used mostly to treat emotional (behavioral) problems.

herbal medicine (also, botanical medicine, phytomedicine, phytotherapy): "the use of plants and plant derivatives as therapeutic agents" (AVMA 1998).

homeopathy: a "medical discipline in which conditions in nonhuman animals are treated by the administration of substances that are capable of producing clinical signs in healthy animals similar to those of the animal to be treated" (AVMA 1998). These substances are usually highly diluted and specially treated medications derived from plant, animal, or mineral sources.

magnetic field therapy: the use of magnets and electrical devices to create controlled magnetic fields, usually applied to specific areas for the treatment of injuries.

naturopathy: a system of medicine using a variety of natural methods to stimulate the body's innate healing capabilities. These methods include diet, herbal medicine, physical therapies, and lifestyle changes.

nutritional medicine: the use of whole foods and nutritional supplementation in the treatment of disease. Nutritional medicine identifies four main influences on nutritional status (Lewith, Kenyon, and Lewis 1996): (1) food quality; (2) food quantity; (3) efficiency of digestion, absorption, and utilization; (4) biochemical individuality.

traditional Chinese medicine: a system of diagnosis and treatment originating in China more than 2,000 years ago, which incorporates diet, exercise, lifestyle changes, indigenous herbs, and acupuncture.

TTouch: a system of circular hand movements applied to the body of an animal; used as a relaxing physical therapy for a variety of species, first described by Linda Tellington-Jones.

Many, many more alternative therapies exist than those defined here. For instance, other native systems, such as the Middle Eastern and South American traditions, provide rich ground for ethnobotanical investigations. Energetic therapies, such as Reiki, Healing Touch, color therapy, and light therapy, may strain credibility, but they find ready acceptance among some veterinary practices and many pet owners. Practitioners who have begun to integrate auxiliary modalities into their practices may want to explore such alternative therapies.

Who Is Using Alternative/Unconventional Medicine?

A major study published in the *Journal of the American Medical Association* described trends in the use of alternative therapies by the American public (Eisenberg et al. 1998). In a nationally representative phone survey conducted from 1991 to 1997, Eisenberg et al. determined that 42.1% of participants had used 1 of 16 alternative therapies. The authors estimated that American health consumers made 629 million visits to alternative medicine practitioners, exceeding all visits to US primary care physicians in 1997. Notably, almost 40% of these consumers never told their physicians they used alternative therapies.

Two interesting surveys were released in 1998 by independent investigators with intriguingly similar results. Haskell with the Stanford Center for Research in Disease Prevention conducted a random telephone survey of 1,000 Americans and inquired about their interest in 19 different modalities, including acupuncture, homeopathy, vitamin therapy, chiropractic, Ayurvedic medicine, Chinese medicine, and other therapies. The study showed that 69% of those surveyed had used some form of complementary and alternative medicine (CAM) in the past year; of those, 55% had somewhat reduced their use of conventional medical services, whereas the rest said their use of CAM did not reduce their visits to their regular doctor. The investigators concluded, "the public doesn't choose between alternative and traditional medicine. Rather, they see the options in a single toolbox and want to choose what works best for them instead of being restricted by arbitrary definitions" (Haskel 1998).

A study reported in 1998 by Kaiser Permanente, the leading US health maintenance organization, indicated that its members were embracing alternative medicine in unprecedented numbers. The study, centered in northern California in 1996, polled 781 physicians and 19,000 members. Ninety percent of the primary care doctors had recommended alternative therapies to their patients, usually chiropractic, acupuncture, massage, and relaxation methods. Nearly 50% of the patient members had tried alternative medicine. Herbs and homeopathy were used by fewer than 10% of the respondents (Gordon, Sobel, and Tarazona 1998).

We do not yet have accurate estimates of CAM use in veterinary medicine, although reasonable conjecture suggests that people interested in CAM might seek to use it in their sick pets. In August 1998, the America Online Veterinary Information Network (VIN) and the Pet Care Forum participated in an Internet survey of pet owners and veterinarians and their interest in complementary and alternative veterinary medicine (CAVM). More than 40% of 1,378 pet owners and 50% of 34 veterinarians stated that they would use complementary therapies as a primary or adjunct treatment; 39.2% of pet owners said they didn't use CAVM because they didn't know enough about it (http://www.vin.com/vinpromo/index.htm). An earlier poll from April 7, 1997, reported that more than 60% of 1,963 pet owners and 380 veterinarians stated that they would use complementary therapies as a primary or adjunct treatment. Interestingly, the 1998 poll received an overwhelming number of comments that suggested that owners believe CAVM is done *without* veterinary advice and is in the realm of home remedies.

Conversely, the 1998 American Animal Hospital Association (AAHA) National Survey of People and Pet Relationships suggested that only 22% of the 1,252 pet owners patronizing AAHA veterinarians had used alternative therapies. Perhaps the wide differences can be explained by different survey populations (Internet surveys may have biased results because respondents are computer-literate, sometimes better-educated consumers). Also, the AAHA survey polled only small-animal pet owners who use veterinary care at AAHA-affiliated hospitals.

In a survey conducted by *Natural Foods Merchandiser* in 1998, pet owners were asked where they purchased herbs and nutraceuticals for their pets. Fully 51% bought these supplements from a health food store, as opposed to 24% who obtained them from their veterinarians. Other sources for "natural" supplements included mail order catalogue (48%), herb stores (19%), and pet stores (10%) (Natural Foods Merchandiser 1998).

Veterinarians are also exploring alternatives. In 1998, the American Holistic Veterinary Medical Association (AHVMA) had grown to include 848 members. The International Veterinary Acupuncture Society (IVAS) had 1,500 members internationally and graduated approximately 100 from certification courses yearly. The American Academy of Veterinary Acupuncture (AAVA), a new organization, had 415 members. The Academy of Veterinary Homeopathy had 120 members (46 certified in veterinary homeopathy) and trained about 35 veterinarians yearly.

Even if only 20% of all pet owners use alternative therapies (which seems like a conservative estimate), the profession is clearly facing a new challenge.

Veterinarians should at least be conversant in these therapies, so they can advise clients on the suitability of the different modalities for their pets or provide referrals to qualified practitioners. For the times when pet owners ask, "Doctor, isn't there anything else you can do?" this book may provide readers with a rudimentary road map for the recommendation of additional therapies—sometimes lifesavers for animals that conventional, proven medicine has failed.

Controversy Surrounding Alternative Therapies

Evidence for Unproven Therapies

Are alternative therapies truly bereft of supporting science? Not really. A practitioner interested in an alternative modality must search a little harder to determine what evidence exists. Some of the stronger herbal, homeopathic, and physical medicine studies are not indexed in Medline, although this situation has improved in recent years. In addition, much of the research on herbal and homeopathic medicine is occurring in countries where these modalities are more heavily used; therefore, some of the best papers may be in foreign languages.

Double Standards

One must be very careful to avoid double standards when assessing evidence for these therapies. That is, beware of requiring a level of research for alternative therapies higher than that for procedures that are already in widespread use. Consider the paucity of supporting evidence for the widely used therapies in the following very limited list:

- Widespread off-label use of antibiotics in food animals
- Low-salt diets, furosemide, propranolol, and procainamide for improving the length of life in dogs with naturally occurring heart disease (Pion 1998)
- Many surgeries
- Phenoxybenzamine to prevent acute reobstruction in cats with LUTD
- Ursodeoxycholic acid in hepatic disease for dogs and cats
- Yearly, triennial, or any other frequency for canine distemper and feline panleukopenia vaccines
- Premium veterinary diet recommendations for improved health
- Most new chemotherapeutics for cancer in most species
- Behavior modification for behavior problems in dogs
- Polypharmacy of the type consistently practiced on older patients

How is progress made in medicine? Scientific support is clearly desirable and allows us to give our patients the best treatments possible. Still, we used aspirin for decades before we knew the mechanism of action, and Jenner's smallpox vaccine was used for close to 100 years before we knew how it worked. There were certainly those who opposed Jenner's work, forming the "Anti-Vaccination League." Estimates of how many conventional medical interventions are well supported by science range from 15% to 80%. If this incomplete proof is true of conventional medicine, shouldn't we be applying the same critical evaluation to every treatment we use?

Still, the literature on alternative medicine is increasing, and one can glean much from even a simple Medline search. Textbooks now exist that attempt to compile the available evidence and describe the rationale behind a therapy and its indications for use. At the end of the day, veterinary practitioners must use intuition, clinical experience, and physiologic rationale as much as they use solid scientific evidence, which exists for only some of their everyday recommendations.

Legal Issues

Herbs and nutritional supplements are regulated, for human use, under the guidelines of the Dietary Supplement Health and Education Act of 1994 (DSHEA). This legislation has come under fire for allowing manufacturers to sell their various wares and for allowing consumers access to untested and potentially dangerous supplements. Recent examples of sales of potentially dangerous dietary supplements have included *Ephedra sinensis*, a sympathomimetic herb used in natural diet pills, and the steroid supplement dehydroepiandrosterone (DHEA). These supplements may have excellent therapeutic qualities when prescribed by a knowledgeable practitioner, but most health food store employees are not so qualified.

DSHEA does not apply to nutraceuticals and plant drugs used in animals. Veterinarians using herbs and dietary supplements are not even prescribing extra-label drugs. In the Extra Label Drug Use, Animal Medicinal Drug Use Clarification Act (AMDUCA) Guidance Brochure supplied by the AVMA, extra-label drug use rules are stated to apply only to approved animal and human drugs. Therefore, the veterinarian is not strictly regulated in prescribing food supplements, but the AMDUCA brochure outlines rules for decision making that might apply. Veterinarians using extra-label drugs or supplements in an off-label manner should consider the following:

1. Make a careful diagnosis within a veterinarian/client/patient relationship (which probably precludes advising unfamiliar pet owners who "just want the dose" for a supplement they just picked up at the health food store!).
2. Determine for a nonfood animal if an approved animal drug exists that contains the needed ingredient, is in the proper dosage form, is labeled for the indication, and is clinically effective. If the answer is yes, use of a dietary supplement may risk scrutiny by authorities.

Many veterinarians considering nutraceutical or herbal supplements are dealing with animals already treated by conventional means without acceptable clinical effect. Using recommendations for extra-label drug use, doctors should keep good records, including the animal name and species, the condition being treated, the established name of the drug, the active ingredient (where known), and the duration of treatment, and should ensure that the drug label is complete, including the veterinarian's name and address, the established name of the drug, directions for use, and cautionary statements.

Conversely, many veterinarians familiar with alternative therapies use them before conventionally recognized treatments or as a viable alternative to them. This practice is undoubtedly because they perceive an improved cost/benefit ratio—the alternative therapies sometimes result in happy, comfortable animals without the adverse effects of some conventional treatments. One example is use of glycosaminoglycan (GAG) supplements for dogs with osteoarthritis before recommending nonsteroidal anti-inflammatory drugs (NSAIDs). Clinical and anecdotal evidence over the last 10–15 years suggests that these supplements are safe and fairly effective, yet the restrictions just described would prevent the use of alternatives in this way. Only now is experimental evidence providing a rationale for using GAGs as a first-line treatment.

The controversy between regulatory authorities and practitioners convinced of the benefits of unproven treatment continues to present problems for all. Maintaining a good doctor/client/patient relationship and discussing *all* options with every pet owner remain the best protection for the doctor using alternatives in medicine.

References

Adverse effects of herbal medicines: An increasing problem? 1998. *Drug and Therapeutic Perspectives* 11(12):14–16.

American Veterinary Medical Association. 1998.Guidelines for Alternative and Complementary Veterinary Medicine. *AVMA Directory and Resource Manual.* 47th ed. Schaumburg, Illinois: AVMA (p. 55).

Angell, M., and J.P. Kassirer. 1998. Alternative medicine—The risks of untested and unregulated remedies. *NEJM* 339(12):839–41.

Brown, L., ed. 1993. *New shorter Oxford English dictionary*, 2 vols. Oxford, England: Clarendon Press.

Chadwick, S. 1999. Veterinarians find alternative cancer treatment for cats and dogs. *Veterinary Economics* 40(5):12.

Eisenberg, D.M., R.B. Davis, S.L. Ettner, S. Appel, S. Wilkey, M. Van Rompay, and R.C. Kessler. 1998. Trends in alternative medicine use in the United States, 1990–1997: Results of a follow-up national survey. *JAMA* 280:1569–75.

Eisenberg, D.M., R.C. Kessler, C. Foster, F.E. Norlock, D.R. Calkins, and T.L. Delbanco. 1993. Unconventional medicine in the United States. *NEJM* 328:246–52.

Gordon, N.P., D.S. Sobel, and E.Z. Tarazona. 1998. Use of and interest in alternative therapies among adult primary care clinicians and adult members in a large health maintenance organization. *West J Med.* 169(3):153–61.

Haskell, W. 1999. Stanford School of Medicine; personal communication.

Lewith, G., J. Kenyon, and P. Lewis. 1996. *Complementary medicine: An integrated approach.* New York: Oxford University Press.

Moore, T.J., B.M. Psaty, and C.D. Furberg. 1998. Time to act on drug safety. *JAMA* 279(19):1571–73.

Natural Foods Merchandiser. 1998. (December).

Pion, P. 1998. Log of the Rounds Room session of October 1st 1998, Veterinary Information Network. Available: http://www.vin.com/members/rounds.

Chapter 2

How to Start

I have little patience for scientists who take a board of wood, look for the thinest part, and drill a great number of holes where the drilling is easy.

—Albert Einstein

Training and Education

Veterinary School Curricula

Veterinary schools teeter on the brink of many changes. Curriculum changes are carefully considered and dearly bought as schools grapple with funding, the need for veterinary participation in biomedical research, and new discoveries in medical science. As a consumer-driven movement and one practitioners have entered as a result of medical need, emerging therapies simply represent a farrago of unrelated modalities to scientists and not a unified group deserving of special study.

Still, burgeoning interest in such therapies as herbal medicine, therapeutic nutrition, and acupuncture has pushed medical and veterinary teachers alike to address this need. More than 50 medical schools offer courses with such titles as "Complementary and Alternative Health Practices" and "Comprehensive Care Case Studies," informal brown-bag lunches, or information within such courses as the "Integrated Clinical Experience." In a recent survey (Wetzel, Eisenberg, and Kaptchuk 1998), 64% of medical schools responding

Table 2.1   American and Canadian veterinary schools that offer CAM courses

School	Course title	Year offered	Instructor
Colorado State University	VM733 Alternative and Complementary Medicine	senior elective	N. Robinson, DVM, DO, G. Ogilvie, DVM, and faculty
North Carolina State University	Introduction to Complementary Veterinary Medicine	years 1–3	H. Berschneider, DVM
University of Florida	VEM 5208 Additional Approaches in Disease Treatment and Prevention	senior elective	R. Clemmons, DVM, PhD, C. Crisman, DVM, MS
Tuskegee University	Course 507 Introductory Veterinary Acupuncture	senior elective	Y.C. Hwang, DVM, PhD
University of Prince Edward Island	VHM 482 Veterinary Acupuncture	senior elective	A. Ortenburger, DVM

offered CAM electives or topics regarding CAM in their required courses. Veterinary colleges are likewise beginning to offer formal instruction in complementary therapies, usually as elective intensives. Except where noted, these courses offer a broad-based introduction to a variety of alternative therapies. Table 2.1 lists those schools currently offering these options.

With the understandable competition for curriculum time, not to mention the awesome and ever-increasing sum of information required to graduate, most doctors gain knowledge of alternative therapies once they enter practice.

Post-Graduate Training

Currently, courses leading to certification (not recognized formally by the AVMA) are offered for acupuncture, chiropractic, and homeopathy (see appendix A). Comprehensive courses in Chinese herbal medicine are also available. Most of these professional-level courses run over 100 hours, involve lectures plus practical experience, and may require continuing education to maintain certification. There is no formal training for veterinarians in nutraceutical therapy, veterinary physical therapy, or Western herbal medicine, though many veterinarians avail themselves of courses in human medicine for these subjects. Certifying organizations are listed in appendix A, along with other organizations related to alternative therapies in veterinary medicine.

Information Access

Fortunately, introductory material may be found fairly easily. Many veterinary conferences offer alternative medicine sessions; for instance, the North American Veterinary Conference offers an entire day assembled by the American Holistic Veterinary Medical Association; the AVMA has offered similar sessions, and many state associations invite speakers trained in these areas.

The American Holistic Veterinary Medical Association has, for more than a decade, sponsored a conference that offers excellent introductory and advanced information on a variety of alternative modalities. More recently, the Midwest and Southeastern Holistic Veterinary Medical Conferences hold two-day seminars covering a variety of treatment modalities. Other weekend courses are often listed in the meetings sections of the *Journal of the AHVMA, JAVMA, DVM Newsmagazine*, and many others.

Until recently, reliable information in book form was sorely lacking. Most books on holistic veterinary medicine were lay-authored and/or directed toward lay audiences. This situation changed with the recent publication of veterinary textbooks on complementary medicine, acupuncture, and Chinese herbal medicine. Table 2.2 lists the most highly recommended textbooks and informal works authored by veterinary experts in alternative medicine. A more complete list of books can be found in appendix B.

Starting in the Absence of Formal Training

The primary purpose of this book is to provide some guidance for veterinarians who wish to get started without formal training. No doubt about it—formal training is vital, but there are reasonably safe and effective treatments that may be used to help patients without spending thousands of dollars on acupuncture or homeopathy training. Veterinarians who use some treatments described in later chapters may be convinced that further investments are, indeed, worthwhile.

Understanding when and how to apply these unfamiliar therapies is often seen as a barrier; many veterinarians have the impression that clients will resist

Table 2.2   Recommended works on alternative medicine

Title	Description
Day, C. 1984. *The homeopathic treatment of small animals: Principles and practice.* Essex, England: The C.W. Daniel Co., Ltd.	An introduction to homeopathic philosophy and suggestions for the treatment of a variety of conditions.
Klide, A., and S. Kung. 1977. *Veterinary acupuncture.* Philadelphia: University of Pennsylvania Press.	This textbook introduces Chinese medicine to the Western professional audience and includes extensive traditional acupuncture point charts.
Pitcairn, R., and S. Pitcairn. 1996. *Natural health for dogs and cats.* Emmaus, Pennsylvania: Rodale Press.	This is a classic handbook of natural therapies written for pet owners. It contains recipes for home-prepared diets and mild herbal, nutritional, and homeopathic treatment suggestions.
Schoen, A. 1994. *Veterinary acupuncture: Ancient art to modern medicine.* Goleta, California: American Veterinary Publications, Inc.	The standard introductory veterinary acupuncture text.
Schoen, A., and S. Wynn. 1997. *Complementary and alternative veterinary medicine: Principles and practice.* St. Louis, Missouri: Mosby-Yearbook.	This is a basic text for veterinarians, introducing philosophy, supporting science, and controversies surrounding a variety of alternative modalities.
Schwartz, C. 1996. *Four paws, five directions.* Berkeley, California: Celestial Arts Publishing.	Although marketed for pet owners, this book is an excellent introduction to traditional Chinese medicine as it relates to health and illness in pets; Five Element Theory; and herbal, nutritional, and physical therapies for a variety of conditions.
Xie, H. 1994. *Traditional Chinese veterinary medicine.* Beijing, China: Beijing Agricultural University Press	Professional-level introduction to traditional Chinese medicine, including herbal prescriptions, acupuncture charts, and protocols for large and small animal species.

Table 2.3   Internet consultations

E-mail lists
Complementary and Alternative Veterinary Medicine List: To apply for a
subscription, contact swynn@emory.edu or jbergeron@monmouth.com.

Bulletin boards
Veterinary Information Network (VIN) maintains the Alternative Medicine Board.
For more information on membership, visit VIN's website at http://www.vin.com.

NOAH, a practitioner board for members of the American Veterinary Medical
Association, maintains an alternative medicine board. For more information on
NOAH, visit the AVMA's website at http://www.avma.org.

unproven therapies. In fact, because surveys indicate that a substantial number
of people are integrating alternatives into their own health care, suggesting the
use of alternative therapies will probably be welcomed by the pet owner.

Owners of pets with chronic problems are especially open to treatment
alternatives. They may feel frustrated, rightly or wrongly, with veterinary medicine in general. Many conditions, such as severe atopic dermatitis or epilepsy,
cannot be controlled without incurring side effects from the required medica-
tion. Owners of animals with malignancies frequently ask for additional alternative medications out of desperation. Chronic conditions are those most often
listed as human patients' reasons for seeking alternatives, and pets with chronic
conditions may be the most likely group on which to become familiar with these
therapies.

Colleagues with experience using herbs or nutritional treatments can be
invaluable sources of information. If one is unfamiliar with local practitioners,
the American Holistic Veterinary Medical Association maintains a referral directory. In addition, there are a number of Internet bulletin boards and e-mail lists
through which one can confer with colleagues on a tough case (see Table 2.3).

Nuts and Bolts of the Holistic Practice

Pricing

Incorporating holistic medicine into a practice changes the schedule for
many a doctor. Because of the extensive history (dietary, environmental, idiosyn-
cratic, etc.) as well as the additional aspects of the physical exam (acupuncture
and chiropractic diagnostics for those trained in these modalities), the consultation takes longer than usual. The first consultation may easily span an hour.

Clearly, pricing structure should reflect these changes. One would predict some resistance in an established practice servicing existing clients; for clients trained to accept the 15-minute consult and a quick fix, the challenge may be insurmountable. Clients who care for pets with chronic problems, however, may welcome a different approach.

Many veterinarians differentiate this pricing structure using specific names like "office call" as opposed to "holistic consultation." Most veterinarians offering these longer consultations will charge significantly more, especially for the first visit. One strategy for determining price is to place a fee proportionate to the time taken for a regular office call. A holistic consultation that takes one hour may cost three to four times the price of the 15-minute office visit.

Space

Many practitioners using these time-consuming intake and treatment procedures have at least one exam room equipped with comfortable chairs and attractive decor. Clients appreciate the relaxed feel and will remember a pleasant experience in the veterinary office.

Role of Staff

Most veterinarians have stood in front of a client who asks, "Doctor, isn't there anything else we can do?" This is the most natural lead-in to a discussion of unproven therapies. Many veterinarians are uncomfortable at this juncture, but pet owners are extremely receptive to the idea of experimental therapies if their pets are still sick, despite all conventional care offers. More often, however, clients begin searching for doctors who offer alternatives to the care they may already have received for their pets, and the front office staff will likely be their first contact.

Reception/First Contact

Not unexpectedly, the Person Who Answers the Phone holds a key role in screening and scheduling the pet owner who wants alternatives. Front office personnel typically encounter two main categories of alternative medicine consumer. The first, and increasingly more common type, is a pet owner who has discovered that "the doctor uses alternative medicine." The receptionist can easily describe the specialized examination and history, ending with the reminder that this significantly longer contact time will cost more than the brief, routine appointment. It is important that the receptionist instruct the new client that all previous records and radiographs are needed at the time of the initial visit.

This type of encounter offers a unique opportunity to develop a referral practice, and like other referral practices, it is advisable to develop good relationships with local colleagues. When the client will allow you contact with their regular veterinarian (and some don't so as not to cause hard feelings), give regular telephone or fax updates, which will be appreciated.

The second sort of caller may be a pet owner who is making an appointment for continued care of a chronic problem, or worse, asking for records to be transferred to a colleague. In this case, the receptionist can mention that the hospital now offers a new service—consultation with a doctor familiar with alternative therapies. Some practices even post reception or exam room signs that read, "If you are using herbs or alternative therapies for your pet, please feel free to discuss this with the doctor."

Technical Support

Technicians may find that the use of alternative therapies in the practice gives them more contact time with clients. They may have more opportunities for client education and perhaps take on an additional role as a physical therapist.

Although the doctor's intake consult takes longer than a standard appointment, client education should get equal emphasis. Many clients need extra contact time to discuss how to monitor results of dietary therapy, how to sleuth out environmental influences on their pet's health, or why they will be reducing the frequency of vaccinations.

Here are a few examples of prepared talks technicians may be giving:

- *General preventive care:* how to choose good commercial diets; how to supplement with fresh food; how to properly prepare homemade diets, etc.
- *Hypoallergenic diet therapy (for allergies, epilepsy, inflammatory bowel disease):* do's and don'ts
- *Weight problems:* how to improve the diet using canned food (because of increased water content) and using vegetables as a substitute for a proportion of the diet; how to break the free-feeding habit, especially for cats
- *Acupuncture:* how much of a time commitment to expect, what adverse effects are possible, etc.

Technicians in holistic practices often become trained in ancillary physical therapies; these might include physiotherapy, massage, and TTouch. These services are often very helpful for patients, and they allow the hospital to provide needed services instead of referring clients to human practitioners or facilities. In addition, technicians can instruct owners in many aspects of physical therapy that can be done at home.

Holistic Practice

Holistic Evaluation

Holistic practitioners are ever cognizant of the totality of a pet's environment. For most veterinarians, this awareness must include a history of the animal's living arrangements, medical problems and treatments, and potential toxic exposures. Doctors using some alternative therapies are obliged to question the owner about more arcane characteristics, such as fears, food preferences, times of day when the condition is worse, and presumed emotional states. For homeopathy and traditional Chinese medicine especially, such a history is vital to making a diagnosis. For the veterinarian prescribing nutraceuticals and herbal drugs in the pharmaceutical model, these questions may still lead to a better understanding of the patient.

Of particular importance are questions about *when* vaccines were given (as opposed to whether "vaccines are current"). If vaccines were given within two weeks to two months of the occurrence of a problem, subsequent vaccines may have to be administered with great care.

Many practitioners ask about pets' diets. If a dog with a skin problem, for instance, is being given a popular commercial diet, many veterinarians assume that the diet is not a problem—all possible nutrients are accounted for—and that further dietary manipulation is unnecessary unless hypoallergenic diets are recommended. Most veterinarians practicing alternative therapies note that pets with a variety of problems who happen to be on standard, easily available, popular diets improve by simply changing to a home-prepared diet or one of a small number of high-quality commercial diets.

Questions about vaccines and diets are the easiest and most basic historical questions. The medical history form in Figure 2.1 suggests many more detailed queries. For instance, if the owner says their dog came from a kennel as a four-year-old retired breeding animal, certain questions about house training are easily understood. If the dog is pruritic only at night, the owner can restrict the use of antipruritic herbs or antihistamines to just before bedtime.

Figure 2.1   Medical history form*

Animal name: _____

Date of birth (month, year): _____

Species: Canine   Feline   Breed: _____

Sex   M   F   Neutered/spayed?   Y   N

Reason for visit today: _____

_____

Where did you get your pet? _____
(pet store, animal shelter/humane society, rescue, breeder,
  stray, or bred in our kennel)?

What sort of "person" is your pet? _____
(nice, moody, nervous, shy but friendly at the same time,
always changing, quick tempered, quick moving, placid)?

Normal diet—explain in detail, including brand of food:

   dry _____

   _____

   canned _____

   _____

   homemade or human food—please list ingredients and proportions _____

   _____

   _____

   snacks _____

   _____

Do you feed free-choice or as meals? How many meals daily? _____

_____

Have you recently switched diets? _____

_____

Any unusual cravings _____
(grass, dirt, bricks, fabric/string, metal, rubber bands, plastic, feces, etc.)?

What are the food and water bowls made of? _____

(continued on next page)

_____

*Partially derived from Richard Pitcairn's homeopathic intake form.

Figure 2.1 Medical history form *(continued)*

List all food supplements (such as vitamins) and herbs currently in use. _____

_____

_____

Does your pet have free access to water? _____

Heartworm prevention type? _____

When was your pet last vaccinated (month and year)? _____

What vaccines were given? _____

What percentage of the time does your pet spend indoors/outdoors? _____

_____

What sort of material is your pet exposed to all day? _____

_____

(dirt, gravel, wool, straw, grass, cedar shavings, carpet, etc.)?

Is your pet in a fenced yard? roaming on acreage? leash-walked only? _____

_____

List all other pets in the home. Do any of them have problems? _____

_____

Have any of them been introduced recently? _____

_____

To what other animals is your pet exposed? _____

_____

(at shows, a groomer's, training classes, friends' homes, etc.)?

Has your pet traveled out of state? When and where? _____

_____

Any major medical problems in his or her history? (List conditions and dates.)

_____

_____

_____

Figure 2.1 Medical history form *(continued)*

Any known food or drug allergies? _____

_____

When did the problem start, and has it changed significantly? _____

_____

Is it a constant problem, or does it occur intermittently? _____

_____

Was there an event in the past that you feel started the problem or that occurred simultaneously? _____

_____

List any changes or problems with the following:

    appetite _____

    activity level, attentiveness _____

    breathing _____

    amount drinking _____

    amount urinating, changes in color or frequency _____

    any vomiting? If so, is it immediately after meals or later? undigested food or

    fluid? _____

    any diarrhea? What does it look like? _____

    coughing? What does it sound like? _____

    sneezing? _____

    any discharges (nose, eyes, ears, vagina, penis, anus, mammary glands)?

        _____

        appearance of discharge: _____

What medications has your pet received for these problems? What was the response?_____

_____

Are the signs constant or intermittent? During what months do you see these signs?

_____

(continued on next page)

Figure 2.1 Medical history form *(continued)*

Are the signs worse at any particular time of day? _____

_____

Is the condition worse or better from, or does animal prefer:

exercise _____

bathing _____

morning, afternoon, evening, late night _____

cold air or heat _____

certain foods _____

eating, drinking _____

emotional upset _____

being touched, pressure _____

excitement/noise _____

Are the signs exacerbated by any particular type of weather (damp, cold, hot, etc.)?_____

Does the problem change site or is it worse on a particular side? _____

_____

Is your pet currently exposed to any of the following?

metals (from paint, enclosures, etc.) _____

dust or fibers (How dusty is the house? What are carpets and rugs composed of?) _____

chemicals (cleaning, finishing, pest control, nearby dumps, etc.)

_____

fumes (from paint, finishes, new carpet, etc.) _____

radiation (any local sources?) _____

Is there a history of exposure to any of the substances just listed? (Please explain any "yes" answers in detail.) _____

_____

_____

_____

Figure 2.1 Medical history form *(continued)*

Are family members also experiencing unusual symptoms? _____

_____

_____

Are symptoms better or worse at home? away from the home environment?

_____

_____

Do you live near an industrial plant, commercial business, dump site, or

nonresidential property? _____

_____

Which of the following do you have in your home? (Circle any that apply.)

    air conditioner, gas stove, wood stove, air purifier, electric stove, humidifier,

    central heating (gas or oil?), fireplace

Have you recently acquired new carpet, refinished furniture, or remodeled your

home? _____

_____

Have you weatherized your home recently? _____

_____

Are pesticides or herbicides (bug or weed killers, flea and tick sprays, collars, pow-

ders, shampoos) used in your home, garden, or on the pet? _____

_____

Do household members have hobbies or crafts? _____

_____

How old is your home? _____

_____

Do you know the history of the home site (long-term pesticide treatments, nearby

landfill sites, etc.)? _____

_____

(continued on next page)

Figure 2.1 Medical history form *(continued)*

Does drinking water come for a private well, city water, or bottled from the grocery store? _____

Complete the remaining questions ONLY if your pet has behavior problems:

When does the animal misbehave (how often and under what circumstances)?

_____

_____

_____

What has been tried so far to correct the problem? _____

_____

Are there any other behavior problems? _____

_____

What is the household schedule on a particular day? Describe a typical day for the animal. _____

_____

Is your dog trained? How obedient would you say she or he is for:

      sit? _____

      stay? _____

      down? _____

      come? _____

      heel? _____

Is he or she equally obedient for everyone in the house? _____

_____

Does he or she obey better in certain places? _____

_____

_____

Who feeds your pet? When and where is he or she fed? _____

_____

_____

Figure 2.1 Medical history form *(continued)*

How does the pet act with

friends? _____

children? _____

strangers? _____

veterinarian? _____

Does your pet have any particular fears (strangers, people, other cats or dogs, other animals, noises, firecrackers, thunderstorms, gunshots, being left alone)?

_____

_____

_____

_____

_____

_____

How does your pet relate to other animals in the house or outdoors?

_____

_____

_____

_____

Is your pet vocal/talkative? _____

_____

_____

Cats:

What types of kitty litter do you use now? _____

Have you tried other types? _____

How often is the box cleaned? _____

Where is it? _____

Is it covered? _____

(Most owners are thrilled when they hear fewer medications are in order.) If an overweight cat prefers dry food, this may lead to the discovery that the owner is feeding free-choice "lite" food in addition to "only feeding ¼ of a small can twice daily"—without satisfactory results.

Many holistic modalities require much more detailed information, however. In Chinese medicine, for instance, certain organ systems are said to be more susceptible to illness at certain times of the year and certain hours of the day. A dog that is pruritic in the front part of the body (neck, front paws) would receive a different herbal prescription from a dog who is more pruritic in the lower abdomen and caudal thighs.

Many of the questions in this form are of use primarily to homeopaths, TCM practitioners, and others using alternative paradigms. The form may still be useful for any doctors to learn more about their patients and about alternative medicine itself.

Stocking the Pharmacy

The object in stocking the pharmacy is to provide clients with supplements that will accomplish the treatment goals. There are now on the market innumerable nutraceutical and herbal food supplements for pets, varying both in strength and quality. Although there are high-quality options available over the counter for common vitamins, such as vitamin E or B-complex, a number of supplements aren't available in consistent form or quality. The veterinarian is left with determining and stocking the remaining supplements; these are an important part of the "alternative" pharmacy.

Quality Control Issues with Herbs and Nutraceuticals

Herbs

Choosing suppliers. Herbal medicines consist of the dried or extracted leaves, roots, stems, seeds, or flowers of plants. Herbs are usually prescribed in dried bulk form, dried extract capsules, alcohol extract tinctures, or glycerin extract tinctures. Practitioners and herbal suppliers should know which preparation provides the most activity, because the active herbal constituents may be alcohol or water soluble but not always both.

Accurate use of the herbal raw material is vital; any herb supplier should be meticulous about making the proper botanical identification and using the appropriate plant parts.

In addition, herb suppliers should obtain their material from known sources, preferably organic or ethically wildcrafted. Pesticides on the plants, for example, could easily remain and become concentrated in the extraction process. Some herbs that are harvested wild have become endangered; goldenseal and ginseng are two very popular examples. Ethical wildcrafters ensure that their harvests leave plants behind for propagation.

Standardized extracts are an increasingly common form of herbal medicine, where one presumably active ingredient is brought to standard concentration in every batch of herb. These preparations are, then, semisynthetic. This practice is controversial among herbalists, who state that seasonal and regional variations in herb composition are part of the art of practice, and that standardization may cause the loss of other equally important herb constituents. In fact, the most effective constituent may not even be known for most herbs.

Caveats for use. These substances have not been tested in companion animals. All dosages are empirical; close monitoring for adverse effects (short term and long term) is highly recommended. Unless otherwise noted, safety during lactation and pregnancy is not established. Unless otherwise noted, doses are proportional to weight, that is, the recommended dose for humans should be used to calculate the appropriate dose for an animal by using the proportion of the animal's weight to a human's weight. A standard dosing table derived from veterinary herbalists using this proportional dosing scheme is provided in chapter 5.

This listing is intended primarily as a resource to help answer client questions about herbs they may be using, but does include herbs with the best potential for clinical use, as well as those with less justification but continued popularity.

Nutraceuticals

Nutritional supplementation is the administration of recognized essential nutrients, such as vitamins or minerals, to ensure that the basic diet is nutritionally replete. Nutraceuticals are dietary supplements that are used for a different purpose. Nutraceuticals have characteristics of both nutrients and pharmaceuticals (Boothe 1997) and may be essential nutrients, nonessential nutrients (such as omega-3 fatty acids and vitamin C for dogs), herbs, organ extracts, and enzymes that are used to treat or prevent disease (Dzanis 1999).

Nutraceuticals may be marketed with a minimum of regulatory supervision (see chapter 1), and the consumer may have little knowledge of the quality control measures used to produce an individual supplement. Briefly, the manufacturer should be using good manufacturing practices (GMP) and should be able to supply a certificate of independent analysis for the product of interest. Ideally, the manufacturer should produce studies supporting that product; these studies are currently few and far between, but ethical companies are beginning to fund more of them. "Good citizens" are companies that support research on their products. Although the products may cost a little more, such companies are worth supporting when they can be found.

Initial Items to Stock the Natural Pharmacy

The pharmacy needn't include every nutritional supplement the doctor will ever use. Vitamin E, for example, is easily found in local grocery stores at a reasonable price. The veterinarian should be more concerned with veterinary-specific products and those products that clients cannot easily find in correct form at local health food stores. Certain patented combination products are often unavailable locally. If the practitioner becomes familiar with such products, stocking them will be a service to pet owners.

Herbs

The following is a list of herbs that may be stocked. (Dosages, indications, and precautions are discussed in chapter 5.)

1. Immunostimulants: astragalus, echinacea, reishi, maitake, others, and their combinations
2. Tonics: ginseng, astragalus, ashwaganda
3. Anti-inflammatory herbs: Boswellia, curcumin
4. Herbs for specific complaints
   - Hepatic: milk thistle
   - Urogenital: cranberry
   - GI: ginger, slippery elm

Nutraceuticals

The following is a list of nutraceuticals that a veterinarian should consider stocking. (Dosages, indications, and precautions are discussed in chapter 4.)

1. Veterinary vitamin-mineral supplement
2. Omega-3 fatty acid supplement (fish oil, flaxseed oil)
3. Antioxidant supplement (for example, Vetri-Science CellAdvance)

4. Glycosaminoglycan supplement (for example, glucosamine sulfate, Cosequin or Glycoflex)
5. Others that may not easily be supplied by local health food stores
    - Vitamins: injectable vitamin C
    - Minerals: vanadium, injectable selenium
    - Amino acids: glutamine, arginine, dimethlyglycine, d-phenylalanine

The First Step: Basic Diet

The cornerstone of practice for veterinarians using natural therapies is dietary manipulation. Concepts of nutritional essentiality as it relates to chronic conditions are rapidly changing. Many veterinarians will manage chronic diseases initially by simply changing or improving the patient's diet and waiting three to four weeks before trying further therapies.

Over the past few decades, the pet food industry has provided convenient and economical foods for domestic animals. Because the public has become comfortable with the idea that commercial pet foods provide complete and balanced nutrition for the life of the animal, basic diet is no longer generally considered an important factor in disease. Pet owners and veterinarians have literally been trained to look elsewhere for causes of disease and treatment options. By ignoring the basic diet when advising pet owners, doctors and retailers are forgetting basic physiological principles: the importance of fresh and varied foods in the diet and biochemical individuality. What consumers in their right minds would believe that food in a bag or can would provide all the nutrition they (personally) would ever need?

Individual Requirements

Dietary recommendations for domestic species have been published in the form of nutrient profiles by the Association of American Feed Control Officials (AAFCO). These nutrient profile recommendations are derived from expert evaluations of National Research Council (NRC) guidelines. The NRC recommendations were based on diets using purified nutrients, assuming 100% bioavailability. AAFCO, an organization composed of state feed control officials, evaluated these recommendations and initiated legislation requiring improved testing and labeling of pet foods (Dzanis 1995). All pet foods must now conform either to AAFCO nutrient profiles or undergo AAFCO-approved feeding trials before being marketed.

These improved procedures do not represent a perfect solution for nutrition of the individual animal, however. In the words of Quinton Rogers, DVM, PhD, one of the AAFCO panel experts, "although the AAFCO profiles are better than nothing, they provide false securities. I don't know of any studies showing their adequacies and inadequacies." Rogers also states that some of the foods that pass AAFCO feeding trials are actually inadequate for long-term nutrition, but there is no way of knowing which foods these are under the present regulations (Smith 1993). This is also true for homemade diets, of course.

Breed and function are important nutritional considerations in domestic animals. For instance, the diets of broiler chickens have had to be revised over time as birds with higher body-weight gain rates were developed (Morris and Rogers 1994). A recent study showed that different breeds of dogs exhibit different abilities to digest the same diet (Zentek and Meyer 1995). Working animals may perform better on (and therefore require) diets high in protein and fat rather than carbohydrates (Kronfeld et al. 1977); diets like these are not commercially available.

Even if our domestic animals were of a homogeneous "race" like their ancestors, as are the wolf, panther, buffalo, and wild horse, they would still display individual differences in physiology and metabolic processes. Biochemical individuality in humans, an area of study pioneered by Roger Williams, applies in many ways to domestic animals. Williams determined that even in normal humans (who are of relatively consistent size and shape), the needs for most nutrients vary over a fourfold range, on average (Williams and Kalita 1977). These factors will vary further according to age, activity level, existing disease, and concurrent drug therapy.

It should be clear that, in addition to uncertainty about the more subtle animal requirements in general, individual animals vary so much in their metabolic function that a blanket recommendation for "any good commercial diet" is a gamble for the pet's health. In general, when we think about how to feed pets, we refer to the "Paleolithic" diet as a starting point. Carnivorous or omnivorous pet animals, like the cat and dog, are presumed to need high-quality meat and fiber sources, along with adequate fat levels, vitamins, and minerals. Interestingly, a requirement for carbohydrates has never been identified in cats, yet commercial dry foods are composed primarily of grains, providing relatively high levels of carbohydrates.

Animals whose individual needs differ due to inbreeding or genetic abnormalities (sometimes common in purebreds) should receive individualized dietary consideration when problems of any sort occur. Each breed, as well as each individual, represents a unique challenge.

Choosing Diets: How to Read a Label

The pet food industry has spent untold millions in formulating diets that provide balanced nutrition in accordance with the AAFCO recommendations, using a variety of basic ingredients. The result is a huge selection of pet foods that occupy a large amount of grocery store shelf space in addition to space in pet stores and health food stores. These foods are often preserved so that nutrient stability may be maintained for a year. The sources of these nutrients and the preservatives used to ensure their extended shelf life may be a problem for some animals.

It has been shown that products with nearly identical guaranteed analyses may have wide variations in digestibility and that cheaper brands are generally not as nutritious (Huber, Wilson, and McGarity 1986). Low-cost ingredients may cause problems related to food intolerance in pets—problems that are easily correctable by using better diets.

Premium diets should contain, at least as the first ingredient, high-quality sources of meat, such as whole chicken, lamb, or meat meals. Whole-grain carbohydrate sources are recognized as superior in human nutrition; however, it isn't unreasonable to assume the same to be true in animal nutrition. The pet food consumer should further investigate *any* ingredient listed, but especially meat by-products and grain fractions (like gluten, mill run, hulls, or dried bakery product). Because animal nutrition science is not perfectly understood, it is possible that whole food sources for micronutrients may also provide as yet unknown phytochemicals or other unidentified conditionally essential nutrients that are necessary for health (Smith and Campbell 1995), despite the fact that AAFCO nutrient profiles don't list them.

To illustrate the difference in quality of various diets, two ingredient listings from actual maintenance-type dry dog foods are presented here. Formula 1 is an easily available national brand, and Formula 2 is a "health food" type brand, in more limited distribution.

- *Formula 1:* Ground yellow corn, soybean meal, meat and bone meal, animal fat (preserved with vitamin E), corn gluten meal, ground wheat, brewers rice, brewers dried yeast, salt, dicalcium phosphate, calcium carbonate, L-lysine, choline chloride, dried whey, wheat germ meal, zinc oxide, ferrous sulfate, vitamin supplements (A, D3, E,

B12), manganese sulfate, niacin, calcium pantothenate, riboflavin supplement, biotin, garlic oil, pyridoxine hydrochloride, copper sulfate, thiamine mononitrate, folic acid, menadione sodium bisulfite complex (source of vitamin K activity), calcium iodate, cobalt carbonate.

- *Formula 2:* Turkey, chicken, chicken meal, whole ground barley, whole ground brown rice, whole steamed potatoes, ground white rice, chicken fat (preserved with natural vitamin E and vitamin C), herring meal, whole raw apples, whole steamed carrots, cottage cheese, sunflower oil, alfalfa sprouts, whole eggs, whole clove garlic, vitamin C (calcium ascorbate), vitamin E supplement, probiotics (freeze dried streptococcus faecium fermentation product, freeze dried lactobacillus acidophilus fermentation product, freeze dried lactobacillus casei fermentation product, freeze dried lactobacillus planturum fermentation product), vitamin A supplement, vitamin D3 supplement, niacin, calcium pantothenate, manganous oxide, vitamin B1 (thiamine mononitrate), vitamin B2 (riboflavin), vitamin B12, vitamin B6 (pyridoxine hydrochloride), vitamin K (menadione sodium bisulfite), folic acid, cobalt carbonate, sodium selenite, biotin.

In this author's experience, animals with GI or dermatologic problems eating Formula 1 very rarely need any treatment beyond switching to something like Formula 2.

Home-Prepared Diets

The profession has historically recommended that owners *never* feed fresh food (or table scraps) to pets. That position needs to be reevaluated now. Some veterinarians now recommend supplementing the diet with meat and vegetables, for carnivores. This practice may provide the pet with phytochemicals (such as bioflavonoids) and other vital nutrients that have yet to be recognized as essential, or even helpful, by nutritional science. The National Cancer Institute has promoted a "five a day" program to encourage *people* to eat five servings of fruits and vegetables a day. This is because studies examining individual nutrients, such as vitamin A or E, have shown that these nutrients alone do not prevent cancer as well as real fruits and vegetables in the diet—and we don't know what is in real foods that works so well. As an example, vitamin E is usually supplied as alpha-tocopherol, because this isomer was found to be "most important." Only recently, other isomers of vitamin E (gamma-tocopherol) and related chemicals (tocotrienols) are receiving attention as having powerful effects. Plant or other whole foods may contain "conditionally essential" nutrients that are beneficial to some sick animals. Is it such a stretch to believe that we also don't know everything about carnivore (or facultative carnivore) nutrition?

An example that may teach us humility about commercial diets comes from a recent paper examining risk factors for "bloat" in large breed dogs; the authors suggest that real food reduces the incidence of this problem (Glickman et al. 1997).

Recipes for homemade diets are easily found; some of the books listed in appendix B are useful. Many veterinarians simply recommend that pet owners use set proportions when preparing a variety of meals. These proportions vary but generally run 25–60% meat (for dogs) up to 80% meat (for cats), 30% carbohydrate source (grain or potato), and 20–45% mixed vegetables. A multiple vitamin-mineral mix and bonemeal or a calcium supplement are recommended as well.

Breed and individual genetic differences may explain why certain pet animals seem to require individualization of the basic diet. Formulas made by major manufacturers keep the majority of pet animals healthy and well, but for animals with problems, the holistic veterinarian will change diets and often discover very basic disease mechanisms easily remedied with food therapy.

Once the patient is getting quality basic nutrition and is prevented from eating preservatives or other potentially problematic chemicals in the daily diet (Dodds 1997), the next step is to consider therapeutic nutrition.

Table 2.4 details three commonly recommended homemade diets.

Table 2.4 Three homemade diets

Poultry Meat and Rice Diet

$1/3$ pound (weight before cooking) poultry
2 cups rice, long-grain, cooked
1 tablespoon sardines, canned, tomato sauce
1 tablespoon vegetable (canola) oil
$1/4$ teaspoon salt substitute—(potassium chloride)
$1/10$ teaspoon table salt
4 bonemeal tablets (GNC 10 grain or equivalent)
$1/5$ multiple vitamin-mineral tablet (made for adult humans)

Analysis: Provides 879 kilocalories, 43.1 grams protein, 37.3 grams fat; supports caloric needs of 29- to 30-pound dog.

Source: Strombeck 1998.

(continued on next page)

Table 2.4 Three homemade diets *(continued)*

Fatty Feline Fare

> 1 cup millet
> 1 egg
> 2 pounds raw chuck roast, hamburger, or roaster chicken with skin
> 3 tablespoons Healthy Powder (Healthy Powder = 2 cups nutritional yeast +
>   1 cup lecithin granules + $1/4$ cup kelp powder + $1/4$ cup bonemeal, or
>   9,000 mg calcium, or 5 teaspoons eggshell powder + 1,000 mg vitamin C)
> $1^1/_2$ tablespoons bonemeal
> 10,000 International Units (IU) vitamin A
> 100–200 International Units (IU) vitamin E
> 1 teaspoon fresh vegetable with each meal (optional)
> 500 milligrams taurine

Directions: Cook millet in 3 cups boiling water, simmering 20 to 30 minutes. Although the recipe does not specify cooking the meat, it could be added during cooking to ensure that enteropathogens are killed. When the millet is soft, stir in egg and rest of ingredients.

Analysis: Yields $7^1/_2$ cups, at about 425 kilocalories per cup.

Source: Pitcairn and Pitcairn 1995.

Hills Lamb and Rice Diet

> $1/4$ pound diced lamb
> 1 cup cooked white rice
> 1 teaspoon vegetable oil
> $1^1/_2$ teaspoons dicalcium phosphate (available at health food stores, or substitute
>   bonemeal)

Also add a balanced supplement that fulfills the canine minimum daily requirement (MDR) for all vitamins and minerals.

Directions: Trim fat from the lamb. Cook (braise or roast) thoroughly without seasoning. Add remaining ingredients and mix well. Keep covered in refrigerator.

Analysis: Protein 7.0%, fat 10.0%, carbohydrate 14.0%, moisture 66.0%, metabolizable energy 795 kilocalories per pound.

References

Basko, I. 1995. Over the counter herbal pet supplements: Fact or fiction? In *Proceedings of the American Holistic Veterinary Medical Association Annual Conference, Snowmass, Colorado.* Bel Air, Maryland: AHVMA.

Berkenwald, A.D. 1998. In the name of medicine. *Annals of Internal Medicine* 128(3):246–50.

Boothe, D. 1997. Nutraceuticals in veterinary medicine: Part I. Definitions and regulations. *The Compendium* 19(11):1248–55.

Dodds, J. 1997. Pet food preservatives and other additives. In *Complementary and alternative veterinary medicine: Principles and practice,* ed. A. Schoen and S. Wynn. St. Louis: Mosby.

Dzanis, D. 1995. The AAFCO dog and cat nutrient profiles. In *Current veterinary therapy XII,* ed. J. Bonagura, 1418–21. Philadelphia: W. B. Saunders.

Dzanis, D. 1999. Interpreting pet food labels—Part 2: Special use foods. *The FDA Veterinarian* 14(6). Available at: http://www.fda.gov/cvm/fda/infors/fdavet/1999/jan.html.

Frank, A.L., and S.J. Balk. 1992. *Case studies in environmental medicine: Taking an exposure history.* Atlanta: Agency for Toxic Substances and Disease Registry. U.S. Department of Health and Human Services.

Glickman, L.T., N.W. Glickman, D.B. Schellenberg, K. Simpson, and G.C. Lantz. 1997. Multiple risk factors for the gastric dilatation-volvulus syndrome in dogs: A practitioner/owner case-control study. *JAAHA* 33:197.

Huber, T., R. Wilson, and S.A. McGarity. 1986. Variations in digestibility of dry dog foods with identical label guaranteed analysis. *JAAHA* 22:571–75.

Kronfeld, D.S., E.P. Hammel, C.F. Ramber, and H.L. Dunlap. 1977. Hematological and metabolic responses to training in racing sled dogs fed diets containing medium, low or zero carbohydrate. *American Journal of Clinical Nutrition* 30:419–30.

Morris, J.G., and Q.R. Rogers. 1994. Assessment of the nutritional adequacy of pet foods through the life cycle. *Journal of Nutrition* 124:2520S–34S.

Pitcairn, R., and S. Pitcairn. 1995. *Natural health for dogs and cats.* Emmaus, Pennsylvania: Rodale Press.

Silver, R. 1999. Practical therapeutics of natural remedies. In *Proceedings of 60th Annual Conference for Veterinarians,* pp. 199–209. Fort Collins: Colorado State University College of Veterinary Medicine and Biomedical Sciences.

Smith, C.A. 1993. Changes and challenges in feline nutrition. *JAVMA* 203:1395–1400.

Smith, S.A., and D.R. Campbell. 1995. The University of Minnesota Cancer Prevention Research Unit vegetable and fruit classification scheme. *Cancer Causes and Control* 6:292–302.

Strombeck, D. 1998. *Home prepared diets for dogs and cats.* Ames: Iowa State University Press.

Wetzel, M.S., D.M. Eisenberg, and T.J. Kaptchuk. 1998. Courses involving complementary and alternative medicine at US medical schools. *JAMA* 280:784–87.

Williams, R.J., and D.K. Kalita. 1977. *A physician's handbook on orthomolecular medicine.* New York: Pergamon Press.

Zentek, J., and H. Meyer. 1995. Normal handling of diets—Are all dogs created equal? *Journal of Small Animal Practice* 36:354–59.

Chapter 3

Sample Protocols

*W*ithout exception, veterinarians using alternative therapies recommend dietary therapy as the first, and primary, treatment. The supplements in the following list will be useful alone; however, working with the pet's diet is vital for two reasons. The first is that subtle dietary inadequacies, dictated by the pet's breed, age, environment, and concurrent conditions, will not often be corrected with single, silver-bullet supplementation. Second, the supplements listed are recommended essentially as drugs, and their long-term safety is untested. If diet changes can ameliorate these disease conditions long term, as many veterinarians have discovered, drug or supplement use can be terminated sooner.

Dietary manipulation is so important that it will be listed repeatedly in the following compendium of conditions as "basic diet." This is not to test the reader's patience, but to remind him or her of the importance of individualized diet recommendations.

The supplements and herbs in the following brief listing are those found helpful in many practices; however, veterinarians who use new and unproven therapies will have diverse opinions on "what works." Those supplements listed appear to help in many cases, but the reader is encouraged to contact colleagues familiar with these therapies for other ideas on individual cases. Treatment principles, where consensus exists, are given in the listing or can be derived from the more detailed information on nutritional supplements and herbs in chapters 4 and 5.

Aging, Disease of

Treatment principles

suppress free radical pathology

immune support, where needed

Best bets

basic diet

B complex

antioxidant vitamins

fish oil/flaxseed oil

Also useful

herbal tonics—ashwaganda, panax ginseng, eleutherococcous, astragalus, codonopsis

Behavior

Anxiety syndromes

kava kava, hops, skullcap, valerian, passionflower

Feline psychogenic alopecia

basic diet (and evaluate for other conditions, such as allergy)

St. John's Wort

Cardiovascular

Congestive heart failure

Treatment principles

control free radical damage from ischemia

support energy metabolism and myocardial function

(In contrast to humans, who commonly require treatments directed toward atherosclerosis and hypertension, dogs and some cats may benefit more from cardiovascular medications that support myocardial function.)

Best bets

basic diet

omega-3 fatty acids (fish/flaxseed oil)

coenzyme Q10

antioxidants

hawthorn—use with caution in hypertrophic cardiomyopathy

Also useful

berberine-containing herbs (Coptis, goldenseal, Oregon grape)

magnesium

Heartworm disease

alternative protocols for treatment using parasiticidal herbs are not recommended, but available

alternative prevention protocols include black walnut and other herbs—not recommended

Digestive

Constipation

Treatment principles

address food intolerances

increase fiber, but with caution in cats with chronic obstipation or megacolon

Best bets

basic diet

vegetable supplementation to basic diet

herbs—psyllium, cascara sagrada, senna, aloe

Diarrhea, nonspecific

Treatment principles

improve GI microbial populations

change fiber levels

address mild maldigestion problems

address food intolerances and allergies

Best bets

basic diet

evaluate for food allergies

probiotics, prebiotics (fructo-oligosaccharides)

fiber: soluble (e.g., psyllium, slippery elm) and insoluble (e.g., vegetables)

digestive enzymes

slippery elm

Inflammatory bowel disease, enteritis

Treatment principles

> address food allergies
> improve GI microbial populations
> decrease intestinal mucosal inflammation and support repair

Best bets

> basic diet; hypoallergenic or elimination diet
> glutamine
> antioxidant vitamins
> omega-3 fatty acids

Also useful

> probiotics and FOS
> herbs: gentian, chamomile, pinellia, slippery elm, boswellia, peppermint

Dental plaque and periodontal disease

> raw meaty bones—this popular alternative dental aid seems to inhibit tartar buildup because of the tearing action required; however, some dogs will fracture teeth on large bones, and GI perforation is a clear risk
> antimicrobial herbs: neem, propolis, myrrh

Marginal gingivitis/stomatitis

Treatment principles

> improve immune function locally and systemically

Best bets

> basic diet
> lactoferrin
> echinacea
> coenzyme Q10

Nausea/motion sickness/vomiting

> basic diet, perhaps hypoallergenic or elimination diets
> ginger, chamomile, peppermint

Pancreatitis

Treatment principles

> reduce free radical damage

Best bets
>
> basic diet
> vitamin C (injectable during acute episodes)
> selenium (injectable during acute episodes)
> vitamin E
> digestive enzymes

Parasites

> pumpkin seed (50% kill of *Dipylidum*)
> garlic, pepper
> berberine-containing herbs (Coptis, Oregon grape) for *Giardia*
> papaya

Ears

Otitis—yeast

Treatment principles
>
> manage underlying allergies

Best bets
>
> basic diet
> vinegar : water (50:50 combination)

Otitis—bacterial

Treatment principles
>
> manage underlying allergies
> suppress microbial growth

Best bets
>
> basic diet
> garlic, mullein

Endocrine

Diabetes mellitus

Treatment principles
>
> lower blood glucose
> increase insulin sensitivity

Best bets
>
> basic diet
> vanadium or vanadyl sulfate
> fish oil

gymnema sylvestre
fiber—soluble and insoluble
panax ginseng
vitamin E

Also useful
arginine
vitamin C
pancreatic glandular

Eyes

Conjunctivitis

Treatment principles
decrease inflammation
control infection, where present

Best bets
cold black or green tea topically
euphrasia tea topically
euphrasia/goldenseal—available commercially

Cataracts

Treatment principles
reduce oxidative damage to lens

Best bets
basic diet
succus cineraria topically
bilberry
vitamin C, E
alpha-lipoic acid

Retinal problems

Treatment principles
reduce oxidative damage to retina

Best bets
basic diet
bilberry
vitamin A

Indolent ulcers

Best bets

  basic diet
  adequan 1:1 in artificial tears
  patient serum

Also useful

  vitamin A
  riboflavin

Glaucoma

  alpha-lipoic acid

Feline herpes keratitis (also see Infectious, feline herpes virus)

Treatment principles

  enhance immune function
  suppress viral replication
  decrease inflammation

Best bets

  basic diet
  lysine

Also useful

  zinc-C 0.25% ocular wash
  riboflavin
  glycosaminoglycan eye wash (may use Adequan injectable)
  patient's serum (spun down and given to the client in a red top
    tube) as a topical treatment for about 3 days
  cold black tea compresses

Hematologic

Hyperlipidemia

  garlic, Guggul

Ischemia/reperfusion

Treatment principles

  reduce oxidative damage

Best bets

  alpha-lipoic acid

Immune Disorders

Immune suppression/Chronic infections

Treatment principles
> enhance immune function

Best bets
> basic diet
> immunostimulant herbs: echinacea, reishi, astragalus, maitake, shitake, ashwaganda, ginseng

Autoimmune disorders, general

Treatment principles
> suppress inflammation, dampen immune reactivity

Best bets
> basic diet
> fish oil
> vitamin E
> DHEA

Infectious

FIV/FeLV

Treatment principles
> enhance immune function
> suppress viral replication

Best bets
> basic diet
> immunostimulant herbs (reishi, echinacea, etc.)
> immunostimulant vitamins: A, C, E
> St. John's Wort

Feline herpes virus/calicivirus URI/stomatitis/keratitis

Treatment principles
> enhance immune function
> suppress viral growth

Best bets
> basic diet
> lysine

immunostimulant vitamins: A, C, E
immunostimulant herbs (reishi, echinacea, etc.)
riboflavin

Integumentary

Alopecia (any breed)

basic diet
melatonin (especially in the boxer, dachshund)

Atopic dermatitis and flea allergy dermatitis

Treatment principles
reduce allergic inflammation

Best bets
basic diet, perhaps hypoallergenic or elimination diets
fish oil
antioxidant vitamins
wash feet for percutaneous sensitizers
vitamin C with bioflavonoids TID

Also useful
bee pollen of local origin
herbs for topical use: witch hazel, aloe, calendula, comfrey,
    chamomile, licorice, Oregon grape

Demodicosis

Treatment principles
enhance immune function

Best bets
basic diet
immunostimulant herbs: reishi, astragalus, etc.
immunostimulant vitamins, especially vitamins E and A

Flea infestation

Treatment principles
eliminate fleas
reduce inflammation secondary to allergic response

Best bets
basic diet

Also useful
>animal: dilute essential oils or infusions of any three of the
>   following herbs: pyrethrum, pennyroyal, citronella, or
>   cedarwood; or powders of diatomaceous earth and pyrethrum
>indoor environment: sodium polyborate powder
>outdoor environment: nematodes, diatom and pyrethrum dusts

Dermatophytosis

Treatment principles
>enhance immune function

Best bets
>basic diet
>immunostimulant herbs: reishi, astragalus, echinacea, etc.
>immunostimulant vitamins: A, E
>topical herbs for isolated lesions: goldenseal

Hyperesthesia, feline

>antioxidants (for steatitis component?)
>St. John's Wort

Burns

Treatment principles
>reduce inflammation
>promote epithelialization

Best bets
>topical herbs: aloe, comfrey, chamomile, calendula, centella
>   asiatica, licorice, honey

Liver

Hepatitis, general

Treatment principles
>reduce inflammation and oxidative damage

Best bets
>basic diet
>vitamin E
>herbs: silybum, cynara, turmeric

Also useful
>glandular or dietary liver (caution with copper content for copper
>   hepatopathy cases)

Hepatic lipidosis
carnitine
arginine
fish oil
zinc
antioxidants

Copper-associated hepatopathy
vitamin C
zinc methionine
vitamin E

Musculoskeletal

Intervertebral disk disease

Treatment principles
reduce inflammation
support disk proteoglycan synthesis

Best bets
basic diet
glycosaminoglycans

Osteoarthritis

Treatment principles
reduce inflammation
support cartilage proteoglycan synthesis

Best bets
basic diet
glycosaminoglycans
refer for acupuncture
DLPA

Also useful
vitamin C
antioxidants
fish oil
boswellia and curcumin combination

Arthritis (rheumatoid)

Treatment principles
reduce inflammation

Best bets
>   basic diet
>   digestive enzymes
>   antioxidant vitamins
>   omega-3 fatty acids (fish/flaxseed oil)
>   elimination diet

Myopathies
>   magnesium
>   carnitine

Trauma
>   bromelain
>   dimethylglycine

Neoplastic

Treatment principles
>   enhance immune function
>   slow tumor growth/metastasis

Best bets
>   diet: homemade, grainless
>   fish oil
>   antioxidant vitamins
>   herbs: garlic, turmeric, maitake, green tea, Essiac (patented
>   combination), carnivora
>   arginine

Neurologic

Epilepsy
>   basic diet, hypoallergenic diet
>   dimethylglycine
>   taurine
>   magnesium
>   melatonin

Senile dementia
>   basic diet
>   gingko

phosphatidylserine
carnitine

Degenerative myelopathy

basic diet
exercise
antioxidants
B-complex
spinal cord glandular
carnitine

Pain, General

DLPA

Respiratory

Asthma, feline

Treatment principles

address allergies
reduce inflammation

Best bets

basic diet, hypoallergenic diet
fish oil
antioxidants
vitamin B6, B12

Feline viral upper respiratory disease (esp. herpes virus)

(see entry under Infectious diseases)

Rhinitis/sinusitis

basic diet
antioxidants
fish/flaxseed oil

Bronchitis, canine

basic diet
bioflavonoids
fish oil
antioxidants

Chylothorax

Rutin

Traumatic

Soft tissue

DMG
bromelain

Urogenital

Chronic renal disease/failure

fish oil
rhubarb (Rheum officinale)
B vitamin or multivitamin-mineral supplement
glandular or dietary beef kidney

Urinary tract infection

cranberry
uva ursi

Feline idiopathic cystitis

Treatment principles

increase water intake to maintain diuresis
reduce mucosal inflammation

Best bets

feed canned or home-prepared diet to increase water intake
glucosamine/glycosaminoglycan supplements
choreito or Polyporus combination

Also useful

antioxidant vitamin
cranberry, if accompanied by infection

Calculi—Oxalate

Treatment principles

diuresis
reduce urinary calcium
reduce mucosal inflammation

Best bets
>   diuretic herbs: parsley, corn silk, dandelion
>   cranberry (reduces urinary calcium)
>   vitamin B6 2mg/kg QD
>   glycosaminoglycans
>   IP-6

Calculi—Struvite

Treatment principles
>   maintain diuresis
>   reduce mucosal inflammation
>   address concurrent bacterial infections

Best bets
>   basic diet
>   cranberry (if accompanied by infection)
>   apple cider vinegar
>   diuretic herbs: dandelion, parsley, corn silk

Prostatic hypertrophy
>   saw palmetto

Chapter 4

Materia Medica of Nutraceutical Supplements

*T*he indications, contraindications, and doses given in the following list are necessarily provisional and experimental.

Algae (blue green algae, spirulina, super green food) *(Kay 1991)*

Actions

protein/amino acid source

carotenoid source

polysaccharide source

Use

stimulates nonspecific immune function (shown in
chickens, mice, etc.)

intense vitamin/mineral/amino acid supplement

anticancer? antiviral?

Contraindications

none described

Adverse effects

may be cyanogenic; has proved toxic in large doses

Dose

proportional to human labeled dose

NOTE: Question mark indicates research may be reported but is scarce or doubtful in conclusions.

Alpha-lipoic acid *(Monograph 1998a; Christopher 1999)*

Actions

antioxidant able to act in fat- and water-soluble tissues

metal chelator

Use

"ideal" antioxidant: diabetic polyneuropathy, cataracts, glaucoma

ischemia-reperfusion injury

Contraindications

none described

Adverse effects

cats have exhibited salivation and ataxia at doses of 30mg/kg BID

Dose

LD_{50} in dogs reported to be 400–500 mg/kg orally

Clinical anecdotes suggest 1–5 mg/kg daily may be safe

Arginine *(Lieberman, Fahey, and Daly 1998; Taboada and Dimski 1995)*

Actions

immune enhancement

inhibits growth of some tumors, prevents tumor formation

improves insulin sensitivity in human obese patients

urea cycle regulation

Use

CHF

cancer

diabetes

hepatic lipidosis, hepatic encephalopathy

Contraindications

none described

Adverse effects

none described

Dose

500–3,000 mg daily

Bioflavonoids (proanthocyanins, e.g., pycnogenol, quercetin, rutin, tea catechins, etc.) *(Franke et al. 1998; Alcaraz and Ferrandiz 1987; Mukhtar, Katiyar, and Agarwal 1994)*

Actions

anti-inflammatory

improves capillary integrity

antioxidant

Use

retinopathy; cataract; conjunctivitis; keratitis (bilberry proanthocyanidins)

many inflammatory diseases, degenerative diseases of aging (pycnogenol from pine bark, tea catechins)

allergy (quercetin, hesperidin)

chylothorax (rutin)

Contraindications

none described

Adverse effects

none described

Dose

proportional to labeled human doses

rutin for chylothorax: 50 mg/kg daily

Carnitine *(Dimski 1995; Kittleson et al. 1997; Furlong 1996; Center 1998; Freeman 1998)*

Actions

integral to energy metabolism

vitamin C–dependent synthesis

Use

heart disease

hepatic lipidosis

weight loss

athletic performance

hepatopathy of American cocker spaniels

senile dementia

Contraindications
>   none described

Adverse effects
>   none described

Dose
>   50–150 mg/kg TID

Carotenoids (lutein, lycopene, beta- and alpha-carotene, xeanthophyllin, and many others)

Actions
>   exogenous antioxidants

Use
>   cancer chemoprevention
>   retinal disorders
>   oxidative stress conditions

Contraindications
>   none described

Adverse effects
>   may cause hypertension in combination with tetracycline in humans

Dose
>   mixed carotenoids (except vitamin A) may be dosed proportionally to
>   human dosage

Chromium *(Spears et al. 1998; Cohn and Dodam 1998)*

Actions
>   essential component of glucose tolerance factor, potentiating activity
>   of insulin
>   may increase insulin sensitivity

Use
>   diabetes mellitus

Contraindications
>   none described

Adverse effects
>   chromium picolinate may be carcinogenic
>   chromium has been implicated in renal nephrotoxicity due to heavy
>   metal overdose

Dose
>   50–300 mcg daily

Coenzyme Q10 (Ubiquinone) *(Rush 1996; Gaby 1996a, 1996b)*

Actions
>   supports energy metabolism as a catalyst in ATP production

Use
>   heart disease—dilated cardiomyopathy, heart failure, etc.

Contraindications
>   none described

Adverse effects
>   rarely, GI effects such as vomiting, diarrhea

Dose
>   may depend on form (powder, oil emulsion, or hydrolysable form)—
>   use per label instructions
>   2.2–20 mg/kg/day

Creatine monohydrate *(Barette 1998; Tarnopolsky and Martin 1999)*

Actions
>   phosphocreatine = ready energy source for muscle function
>   promotes protein/muscle synthesis

Use
>   athletic performance
>   neuromuscular diseases
>   geriatric muscle wasting?

Contraindications
>   renal disease

Adverse effects
>   none reported

Potential interactions

    cimetidine, trimethoprim, probenicid

Dose

    label dose on veterinary products

Dehydroepiandrosterone (DHEA) *(MacEwen and Kurzman 1991; Regelson and Kalimi 1994; Regelson, Loria, and Kalimi 1994; Gaby 1996c)*

Actions

    adrenal steroid precursor

Use

    diseases of aging?
    autoimmune disorders, especially lupus
    obesity?

Contraindications

    liver disease

Adverse effects

    may cause hepatitic abnormalities

Dose

    5–50 mg daily

Dimethylglycine (DMG) *(Roach and Carlin 1982; Graber et al. 1981; Weiss 1992; Seiler and Sarhan 1984)*

Actions

    may decrease lactic acid accumulation during exercise
    may enhance immune response (shown in humans, rabbits, and
       mice; disputed in cats)
    anticonvulsant-glycine receptor agonist in CNS

Use

    to reduce seizure frequency in epilepsy

Contraindications

    none described

Adverse effects

    nontoxic

Dose

50–400 mg daily

Enzymes (proteolytic) *(Stauder, Pollinger, and Fruth 1990; Batkin, Taussig, and Szekeres 1988; Nakazawa, Emancipator, and Lamm 1986; Monograph 1998b)*

Actions

anti-inflammatory
anticoagulant? (bromelain)
antimetastatic? (bromelain)

Use

exocrine pancreatic insufficiency (EPI)
chronic inflammatory disease—especially involving immune complex
disease
musculoskeletal trauma

Contraindications

none described

Adverse effects

may cause some gastritis and vomiting

Dose

veterinary products such as Prozyme, Vetzyme, or Viokase: labeled
dose
bromelain: proportional to human label dose

Fiber *(Nelson et al. 1998; Gray 1995; Spiller 1994)*

Actions

soluble (pectin, guar gum, psyllium, slippery elm): stool softening,
bulking, slows glucose absorption from small intestine
insoluble (cellulose, peanut hulls, soy mill run): stool softening,
bulking
mixed soluble and insoluble (soy fiber, beet pulp, pea fiber)
lignan (flaxseed): anti-estrogenic activity

Use

constipation
diabetes mellitus

hyperlipidemia

diarrhea, especially of inflammatory bowel disorders or colitis

Contraindications

colonic obstruction

dehydration

Adverse effects

loose stool, increased defecation

Dose

veterinary products (such as Vetasyl) as labeled

proportionate to human dose

Glutamine *(Griffiths 1997; Elia and Lunn 1997; Newsholme and Calder 1997)*

Actions

promotes/maintains mucosal healing in the gut

protein sparing in catabolic states

supports immune function

Use

inflammatory bowel disease, colitis

muscle wasting, chronic debilitating disease

immunostimulant

Contraindications

none described

Adverse effects

none described

Dose

0.5 g/kg per day (divided as necessary)

Glyconutritionals (Acemannan, Ambrotose) *(Axford 1997)*

Actions

mediates cell communication?

Use

immune stimulation

cancer

Contraindications
>   none described

Adverse effects
>   none described

Dose
>   proportionate to human dose

Sulfated glycosaminoglycans and precursors (Chondroitin sulfate, pentosan polysulfate, glucosamine HCL, glucosamine sulfate) *(McNamara, Johnston, and Todhunter 1997; Hwang et al. 1997)*

Actions
>   cartilage constituent
>   present in bladder mucosa, vascular endothelium, etc.

Use

>   osteoarthritis
>   rheumatoid arthritis
>   wound healing
>   feline idiopathic cystitis (IC)

Contraindications
>   contraindicated in presence of coagulopathy

Adverse effects
>   mild GI upset with vomiting and diarrhea

Dose
>   veterinary forms (such as Cosequin) as labeled for arthritis
>   proportionate to human label dose
>   pentosan polysulphate for feline IC: 8 mg/kg BID

IP-6 (inositol hexaphosphate) *(Shamsuddin, Vucenik, and Cole 1997)*

Actions
>   controls cell division
>   increases natural killer cytotoxicity?
>   antioxidant

Use

>   tumors, especially carcinomas (liver, lung, breast, colon, skin) and
>   leukemias

Contraindications
> none described

Adverse effects
> none reported

Dose
> 25–100 mg/kg, based on human and laboratory animal studies

Lactoferrin *(Sato et al. 1996)*

Actions
> binds iron ions essential to bacterial growth
> immune modulator

Use
> feline stomatitis

Contraindications
> none described

Adverse effects
> none described

Dose
> 40 mg/kg topically (mixed in milk, syrup)

Lysine (Collins, Nasisse, and Moore 1995; Nasisse 1998)

Actions
> adequate or higher blood levels may suppress herpesviral
> replication

Use
> feline recurrent herpesvirus infection—upper respiratory signs or
> keratitis

Contraindications
> none described

Adverse effects
> none reported

Dose

250–500 mg mixed in food daily

Magnesium *(Martin, Van Pelt, and Wingfield 1995; Dhupa 1995; Autran de Morais and Hansen 1995)*

Actions

integral to bone, protein, and fat formation
cellular and metabolic functions, especially in energy production
involved in clotting function, B vitamin activity, insulin function, regulation of vascular smooth muscle tone

Use

cardiovascular disease
neurologic disorders
small intestinal disease
diabetes mellitus
chronic debilitating disease and hospitalization

Contraindications

renal disease

Adverse effects

hypocalcemia, hypotension, respiratory depression, cardiac arrest when administered intravenously

Potential interactions

furosemide, phenobarbital, phenytoin, and tetracycline may cause malabsorption
hydrochlorthiazide depletes magnesium levels

Dose

5 mg/lb p.o. daily

Melatonin *(Hughes, Sack, and Lewy 1998; Bartsch and Bartsch 1997; Lamberg 1996; Molina-Carballo et al. 1997)*

Actions

regulates circadian clock; induces sleep
antioxidant

Use
> senile insomnia
> some cancers
> epilepsy?
> alopecia in some short-haired breeds

Contraindications
> none described

Adverse effects
> mild hypothermia? possible suppression of male fertility?

Dose
> 1–5 mg before bed
> for alopecia in boxers, 6 mg TID

Omega-3 fatty acids (fish oil, flaxseed oil) *(Ogilvie et al. in press; Brown et al. 1998; Burke, Lichtenstein, and Rombeau 1997; Singh, Hamid, and Reddy 1997; Schut et al. 1997; Leaf and Kang 1996; Gogos et al. 1998; Hall et al. 1999; Freeman et al. 1998)*

Actions
> modulates eicosanoid production
> induces cell differentiation and apoptosis
> ameliorates insulin resistance
> may reduce CD4:CD8 lymphocyte ratio

Use
> cancer
> diabetes mellitus
> chronic renal disease
> many inflammatory diseases (inflammatory bowel disease, atopic
>   dermatitis, rheumatoid arthritis, lupus)
> cardiovascular disease

Contraindications
> coagulopathy?

Adverse effects
>   may interfere with clotting

Dose
>   60–100 mg/kg

dl-phenylalanine (DLPA) *(Budd 1983; Kitade et al. 1988)*

Actions
>   precursor to L-dopa, NE, epinephrine
>   inhibits decarboxylation of endogenous opioids

Use
>   pain (especially arthritic)
>   may enhance acupuncture analgesia

Contraindications
>   none described

Adverse effects
>   none described

Dose
>   250–500 mg BID

Phosphatidylserine *(Kidd, 1996)*

Actions
>   membrane phospholipid, which facilitates signal transduction

Use
>   senile cognitive dysfunction

Contraindications
>   none described

Adverse effects
>   none described; dogs tolerated 70 gm/day in one study

Dose
>   100–500 mg daily

Probiotics and fructo-oligosaccharides *(Drago et al. 1997; Sparkes et al. 1998; Schiffrin et al. 1997; Willard 1996)*

Actions

competitive inhibition of enteropathogens

may modulate neuropeptide levels

may improve athletic performance in race horses

may improve weight gain in pigs and mice

Use

IBD

food allergy

immune suppression

diarrhea

chronic antibiotic use

Contraindications

none described

Adverse effects

none reported

Dose

as labeled, or proportional; some are using much higher doses
successfully

Propolis *(de Campos et al. 1998; Miyataka et al. 1998; Steinberg, Kaine, and Gedalia 1996; Takaisi-Kikuni and Schilcher 1994; Basnet, Matsuno, and Neidlein 1997; Mirzoeva and Calder 1996)*

Actions

antimicrobial

anti-inflammatory

antioxidant

analgesic

may inhibit histamine release

Use

periodontal infections

other bacterial infections

liver damage
allergy

Contraindications
none described

Adverse effects
rare contact dermatitis

Dose
aqueous preparation as a dental rinse
orally, proportionate to human dose

Selenium *(Clark et al. 1996; Kraft et al. 1995)*

Actions
integral to antioxidant functions of glutathione peroxidase and
vitamin E

Use
pancreatitis
cancer prevention
cardiovascular disease

Contraindications
none described

Adverse effects
alkali disease and blind staggers are well described in large animals
reported minimum lethal dose in dogs: 2 mg/kg IM—may cause
acute death at this level

Dose
5–50 mcg daily
0.3 mg/kg sodium selenite intravenously for acute pancreatitis

Superoxide dismutase (S.O.D.)

Actions
endogenous antioxidant enzyme

Use

> osteoarthritis
> heart disease

Contraindications

> none described

Adverse effects

> none reported

Dose

> 5–20 IU/kg; not well explored yet

Taurine *(Birdsall 1998; Kittleson et al. 1997; Center 1998; Freeman 1998)*

Actions

> bile acid conjugation
> membrane stabilization
> modulates cellular calcium levels

Use

> cardiac disorders, especially for dilated cardiomyopathy of cats and
>   American cocker spaniels
> liver disease
> epilepsy

Contraindications

> none described

Adverse effects

> none reported

Dose

> 500 mg TID is recommended for cocker spaniels with dilated
>   cardiomyopathy
> 250–500 mg BID is recommended for cats

Vanadium *(Verma, Cam, and McNeill 1998; Greco 1997)*

Actions
>enhances insulin sensitivity
>post–insulin receptor glucose metabolism activator
>reduces pancreatic insulin depletion

Use
>diabetes mellitus

Contraindications
>none described

Adverse effects
>anorexia, vomiting—usually transient

Dose
>vanadium 0.2 mg/kg QD or vanadyl sulfate 1 mg/kg QD

Vitamin C (ascorbic acid, sodium ascorbate, magnesium ascorbate, Ester-C) *(Plumb 1999)*

Actions
>antioxidant
>integral to collagen formation
>antihistamine-like action
>may support immune function

Use
>allergy
>chronic inflammatory disorders
>cancer
>cataracts
>gingivitis
>immune enhancement
>endothelial dysfunction in CV/ischemic disorders

Contraindications
>none described

Adverse effects

> gastritis and diarrhea occur consistently at high doses—start at low
> end of dose and increase gradually

Potential interactions

> tetracyclines deplete vitamin C
> salicylates deplete vitamin C
> vitamin C may interfere with action of aminoglycosides in urine

Dose

> 50 mg/kg, up to 1,000 mg/day in large dogs
> Doses of 3–5 g per day have been used without adverse effect in large
> dogs

Vitamin E *(Twedt et al. 1998; Meydani et al. 1998; Werbach 1997:158)*

Actions

> fat-soluble membrane stabilizer

Use

> cholestatic liver disease
> humans: prevents cardiovascular disease
> diabetes
> inflammatory disorders
> epilepsy
> immune modulator
> intervertebral disk disease

Contraindications

> none described

Adverse effects

> rare GI disturbances
> may exacerbate hypertension?

Potential interactions

> in combination with digoxin, may cause hypercalcemia and
> arrhythmias

Dose

    10–20 IU/kg, up to 800 IU daily for large dogs

Zinc *(Scott, Miller, and Griffin 1995:238; Plumb 1999)*

Actions

    enzyme system co-factor

Uses

    zinc-responsive dermatoses of huskies and malamutes
    immune support
    toenail abnormalities
    retinal abnormalities

Contraindications

    none described

Adverse effects

    gastritis
    large doses can cause hemolytic anemia, icterus, hypotension

Potential interactions

    furosemide, penicillamine, and tetracyclines cause malabsorption
    hydrochlorthiazide may deplete zinc levels
    large doses inhibit copper storage

Dose

    zinc methionine 4 mg/kg daily p.o.
    zinc sulfate 10 mg/kg daily p.o.
    zinc gluconate 5 mg/kg daily p.o.

References

Alcaraz, M.J., and M.L. Ferrandiz. 1987. Modification of arachidonic metabolism by flavonoids. *J Ethnopharmacol* 21(3):209–29.

Autran de Morais, H.A., and B. Hansen. 1995. Chloride and magnesium: The forgotten ions. In *Proceedings of the 13th ACVIM Forum, Lake Buena Vista, Florida*, pp. 628–31. Lakewood, Colorado: ACVIM.

Axford, J. 1997. Glycobiology and medicine: An introduction. *J Royal Soc Med* 90:260–64.

Barette, E.P. 1998. Creatine supplementation for enhancement of athletic performance. *Alternative Medicine Alert* 1(7):73–84.

Bartsch, C., and H. Bartsch. 1997. Significance of melatonin in malignant diseases. *Wien Klin Wochenschr* 109(18):722–29.

Basnet, P., T. Matsuno, and R. Neidlein. 1997. Potent free radical scavenging activity of propol isolated from Brazilian propolis. *Z Naturforsch* 52(11–12):828–33.

Batkin, S., S.J. Taussig, and J. Szekeres. 1988. Antimetastatic effect of bromelain with or without its proteolytic and anticoagulant activity. *J Cancer Res Clin Oncol* 114:507–8.

Birdsall, T.C. 1998. Therapeutic applications of taurine. *Alternative Medicine Review* 3(2):128–36.

Brown, S.A., C.A. Brown, W.A. Crowell, J.A. Barsanti, T. Allen, C. Cowell, and D.R. Finco. 1998. Beneficial effects of chronic administration of dietary ω-3 fatty acids in dogs with renal insufficiency. *Journal of Laboratory and Clinical Medicine* 131:447–54.

Budd, K. 1983. Use of D-phenylalanine, an enkephalinase inhibitor, in the treatment of intractable pain. *Advances in Pain Research and Therapy* 5:305–8.

Burke, A., G.R. Lichtenstein, and J.L. Rombeau. 1997. Nutrition and ulcerative colitis. *Baillieres Clin Gastroenterol* 11(1):153–74.

Bushman, J.L. 1998. Green tea and cancer in humans: A review of the literature. *Nutrition and Cancer* 31(3):151–59.

Center, S.A. 1998. Nutritional support for dogs and cats with hepatobiliary disease. *J Nutr.* 128:2733S–46S.

Christopher, M. 1999. Personal communication. Department of Pathology, Microbiology and Immunology, School of Veterinary Medicine, University of California, Davis.

Clark, L.C., G.F. Combs, B.W. Turnbull, E.H. Slate, D.K. Chalker, J. Chow, L.S. Davis, R.A. Clover, G.F. Graham, E.G. Gross, A. Knograd, J.L. Lesher, H.K. Park, B.B. Sanders, C.L. Smith, and J.R. Taylor. 1996. Effects of selenium supplementation for cancer prevention in patients with carcinoma of the skin. *JAMA* 276(24):1957–85.

Cohn, L.A., and J.R. Dodam. 1998. Effect of chromium on glucose tolerance in normal-weight and obese cats. Abstract No. 169. *JACVIM* 12(3):240.

Collins, K., M. Nasisse, and C. Moore. 1995. In vitro efficacy of L-lysine against feline herpesvirus type-1. In *Proceedings of the American College of Veterinary Ophthalmology*, p. 141 Newport, Rhode Island: ACVO.

de Campos, R.O., N. Paulino, C.H. da Silva, A. Scremin, and J.B. Calixto. 1998. Anti-hyperalgesic effect of an ethanolic extract of propolis in mice and rats. *J Pharm Pharmacol* 50(10):1187–93.

Dhupa, N. 1995. Magnesium therapy. In *Current veterinary therapy XII: Small animal practice*, ed. J. Bonagura, pp. 132–33. Philadelphia: W. B. Saunders.

Dimski, D.S. 1995. Carnitine supplementation in treatment of hepatic lipidosis in cats. In *13th ACVIM Forum Proceedings*. Lakewood, Colorado: ACVIM.

Drago, L., M.R. Gismondo, A. Lombardi, C. de Haen, and L. Gozzini. 1997. Inhibition of in vitro growth of enteropathogens by new *Lactobacillus* isolates of human intestinal origin. *FEMS Microbiol Lett* 153(2):455–63.

Elia, M., and P.G. Lunn. 1997. The use of glutamine in the treatment of gastrointestinal disorders in man. *Nutrition* 13(7–8):743–47.

Franke, A.A., R.V. Cooney, L.J. Custer, L.J. Mordan, and Y. Tanaka. 1998. Inhibition of neoplastic transformation and bioavailability of dietary flavonoid agents. *Adv Exp Med Biol* 439:237–48.

Freeman, L.M. 1998. Interventional nutrition for cardiac disease. *Clin Tech Small Anim Pract* 13:232–37.

Freeman, L.M., J.E. Rush, J.J. Kehayias, J.N. Ross, S.N. Meydani, D.J. Brown, G.G. Dolnikowski, B.N. Marmor, M.E. White, C.A. Dinarello, and R. Roubenoff. 1998. Nutritional alterations and the effect of fish oil supplementation in dogs with heart failure. *J Vet Intern Med* 12(6):440–48.

Furlong, J.H. 1996. Acetyl-L-carnitine: Metabolism and applications in clinical practice. *Alternative Medicine Review* 1(2):85–93.

Gaby, A.R. 1996a. The role of coenzyme Q10 in clinical medicine: Part 1. *Alternative Medicine Review* 1(1):11–17.

Gaby, A.R. 1996b. The role of coenzyme Q10 in clinical medicine: Part II. *Alternative Medicine Review* 1(3):168–75.

Gaby, A.R. 1996c. Dehydroepiandrosterone: Biological effects and clinical significance. *Alternative Medicine Review* 1(2):60–69.

Gogos, C.A., P. Ginopoulos, B. Salsa, E. Apostolidou, N.C. Zoumbos, and F. Kalfarentzos. 1998. Dietary omega-3 polyunsaturated fatty acids plus vitamin E restore immunodeficiency and prolong survival for severely ill patients with generalized malignancy: A randomized control trial. *Cancer* 82(2):395–402.

Graber, C.D., J.M. Goust, A.D. Glassman, R. Kendall, and C.B. Loadholt. 1981. Immunomodulating properties of dimethylglycine in humans. *J Infect Dis* 143(1):101–5.

Gray, D.S. 1995. The clinical uses of dietary fiber. *American Family Physician* 51(2):419–25.

Greco, D.S. 1997. Treatment of noninsulin-dependent diabetes mellitus with oral hypoglycemic agents. In *Proceedings of the 15th ACVIM Forum, Lake Buena Vista, Florida*, p. 252. Lakewood, Colorado: ACVIM.

Griffiths, R.D. 1997. Outcome of critically ill patients after supplementation with glutamine. *Nutrition* 13(7–8):752–54.

Hall, J.A., R.C. Wander, J.L. Gradin, S.H. Du, and D.E. Jewell. 1999. Effect of dietary n-6 to n-3 ratio on complete blood and total white blood cell counts, and T-cell subpopulations in dogs. *AJVR* 60(3):319–27.

Hughes, R.J., R.L. Sack, and A.J. Lewy, 1998. The role of melatonin and circadian phase in age-related sleep-maintenance insomnia: Assessment in a clinical trial of melatonin replacement. *Sleep* 21(1):52–68.

Hwang, P., B. Auclair, D. Beechinor, M. Diment, and T.R. Einarson. 1997. Efficacy of pentosan polysulfate in the treatment of interstitial cystitis: A meta-analysis. *Urology* 50(1):39–43.

Kay, R.A. 1991. Microalgae as food and supplement. *Critical Reviews in Food Science and Nutr.* 30(6):555–73.

Kidd, P.M. 1996. Phosphatidylserine: Membrane nutrient for memory. A clinical and mechanistic assessment. *Alternative Medicine Review* 1:70–84.

Kitade, T., Y. Odahara, S. Shinohara, T. Ikeuchi, T. Sakai, K. Morikawa, M. Minamikawa, S. Toyota, A. Kawachi, M. Hyodo, and E. Hosoya. 1988. Studies on the enhanced effect of acupuncture analgesia and acupuncture anesthesia by D-phenylalanine (first report)—effect on pain threshold and inhibition by naloxone. *Acupunct. Electrother. Res* 13(2–3):87–97.

Kittleson, M.D., B. Keene, P.D. Pion, C.G. Loyer, and the MUST Study Investigators. 1997. Results of the Multicenter Spaniel Trial (MUST): Taurine- and carnitine-responsive dilated cardiomyopathy in American cocker spaniels with decreased plasma taurine concentration. *J Vet Intern Med* 11(4):204–11.

Kraft, W., A. Kaimaz, M. Kirsch, and A. Hoerauf. 1995. Behandlung akuter pankreatiden des hundes mit selen. *Kleintierpraxis* 40:35–43.

Lamberg, L., 1996. Melatonin potentially useful but safety, efficacy remain uncertain. *JAMA* 276(3):1011–14.

Leaf, A., and J.X. Kang. 1996. Prevention of cardiac sudden death by N-3 fatty acids: A review of the evidence. *J Internal Medicine* 240:5–12.

Lieberman, E.D., T.J. Fahey, and J.M. Daly. 1998. Immunonutrition: The role of arginine. *Nutrition* 14(7–8):611–17.

MacEwen, E.G., and I.D. Kurzman. 1991. Obesity in the dog: Role of the adrenal steroid dehydroepiandrosterone (DHEA). *J Nutr Nov* 121:11, Suppl S51–55.

Martin, L.G., D.R. Van Pelt, and W.E. Wingfield. 1995. Magnesium and the critically ill patient. In *Current veterinary therapy XII: Small animal practice*, ed. J. Bonagura, pp. 128–31. Philadelphia: W. B. Saunders.

McNamara, P.S., S.A. Johnston, and R.J. Todhunter. 1997. Slow-acting, modifying agents. *Veterinary Clinics of North American, Small Animal Practice* 27(4):863–67, 951–52.

Meydani, S.N., M.G. Hayek, D. Wu, and M. Meydani. 1998. Vitamin E and immune response in aged dogs. In *Iams Nutrition Symposium Proceedings*, pp. 295–303. Vol. 2, *Recent advances in canine and feline nutrition*. Wilmington Ohio: Orange Frazer Press.

Mirzoeva, O.K., and P.C. Calder. 1996. The effect of propolis and its components on eicosanoid production during the inflammatory response. *Prostaglandins Leukot Essent Fatty Acids* 55(6):441–49.

Miyataka, H., M. Nishiki, H. Matsumoto, T. Fujimoto, M. Matsuka, A. Isobe, and T. Satoh. 1998. Evaluation of propolis (II): Effects of Brazilian and Chinese propolis on histamine release from rat peritoneal mast cells induced by compound 48/80 and concanavalin A. *Biol Pharm Bull* 21(7):723–29.

Molina-Carballo, A., A. Munoz-Hoyos, R.J. Reiter, M. Sanchez-Forte, F. Moreno-Madrid, M. Rufo-Campos, J.A. Molina-Font, and D. Acuna-Castroviejo. 1997. Utility of high doses of melatonin as adjunctive anticonvulsant therapy in a child with severe myoclonic epilepsy: Two years' experience. *J Pineal Res* 23(2):97–105.

Monograph: Alpha-lipoic acid. 1998a. *Alternative Medicine Review* 3(4):308–10.

Monograph: Bromelain. 1998b. *Alternative Medicine Review* 3(4):302–5.

Mukhtar, H., S.K. Katiyar, and R. Agarwal. 1994. Cancer chemoprevention by green tea components. *Adv Exp Med Biol* 354:123–34.

Nakazawa, M., S.N. Emancipator, and M.E. Lamm. 1986. Proteolytic enzyme treatment reduces glomerular immune deposits and proteinuria in passive Heymann nephritis. *J Exp Med* 164:1973–87.

Nasisse, M.P. 1998. *114th Ohio VMA Conference: Feline Ophthalmology—Part I.* Columbus, Ohio: OVMA.

Nelson, R.W., C.A. Duesberg, S.L. Ford, E.C. Feldman, D.J. Davenport, C. Kiernan, and L. Neal. 1998. Effect of dietary insoluble fiber on control of glycemia in dogs with naturally acquired diabetes mellitus. *JAVMA* 212:380–89.

Newsholme, E.A., and P.C. Calder. 1997. The proposed role of glutamine in some cells of the immune system and speculative consequences for the whole animal. *Nutrition* 13(7–8):728–30.

Ogilvie, G.K., M.J. Fettman, C.H. Mallinckrodt, J.A. Walton, R.A. Hansen, D.J. Davenport, K.L. Gross, K.L. Richardson, Q. Rogers, and M.S. Hand. In press. Effect of fish oil and arginine on remission and survival in dogs with lymphoma: A double blind, randomized study. *Cancer.*

Plumb, D.C., 1999. *Veterinary drug handbook.* 3rd ed. Ames: Iowa State University.

Regelson, W., and M. Kalimi. 1994. Dehydroepiandrosterone (DHEA)—the multifunctional steroid. Part 2, Effects on the CNS, cell proliferation, metabolic and vascular, clinical and other effects. Mechanism of action? *Ann N Y Acad Sci* 719:564–75.

Regelson, W., R. Loria, and M. Kalimi. 1994. Dehydroepiandrosterone (DHEA)—the "mother steroid." Part 1, Immunologic action. *Ann N Y Acad Sci* 719:553–63.

Roach, E.S., and L. Carlin. 1982. N, N-dimethylglycine for epilepsy (letter). *NEMJ* 307(17):1081–82.

Rush, J.E. 1996. Alternative therapies for heart failure patients. In *Proceedings of the 14th Annual Conference of the American College of Veterinary Internal Medicine, May 23–26, San Antonio.* Lakewood, Colorado: ACVIM.

Sato, R., O. Inanami, Y. Tanaka, M. Takase, and Y. Naito. 1996. Oral administration of bovine lactoferrin for treatment of intractable stomatitis in feline immunodeficiency virus (FIV)-positive and FIV-negative cats. *Am J Vet Res* 57(10):1443–46.

Schiffrin, E.J., D. Brassart, A.L. Servin, F. Rochat, and A. Donnet-Hughes. 1997. Immune modulation of blood leukocytes in humans by lactic acid bacteria: Criteria for strain selection. *Am J Clin Nutr* 66:2:515S–20S.

Schut, H.A., C.L. Wang, L.M. Twining, and K.M. Earle. 1997. Formation and persistence of DNA adducts of 2-amino-3-methylimmidazol[4,5-f]quinoline (IQ) in CDF1 mice fed a high omega-3 fatty acid diet. *Mutat Res* 378(1–2):23–30.

Scott, D.W., W.H. Miller, and C.E. Griffin. 1995. Dermatologic therapy. In *Small animal dermatology.* 5th ed. Philadelphia: W.B. Saunders Co.

Seiler, N., and S. Sarhan. 1984. Synergistic anticonvulsant effects of GABA-T inhibitors and glycine. *Naunyn Schmiedebergs Arch Pharmacol* 326(1):49–57.

Shamsuddin, A.M., I. Vucenik, and K.E. Cole. 1997. IP6: A novel anti-cancer agent. *Life Sci* 61(4):343–54.

Singh, J., R. Hamid, and B.S. Reddy. 1997. Dietary fat and colon cancer: Modulation of cyclooxygenase-2 by types and amount of dietary fat during the postinitiation stage of colon carcinogenesis. *Cancer Res* 57(16):3465–70.

Sparkes, A.H., K. Papasouliotis, G. Sunvold, G. Werrett, E.A. Gruffydd-Jones, K. Egan, T.J. Gruffydd-Jones, and G. Reinhart. 1998. Effect of dietary supplementation with fructo-oligosaccharides on fecal flora of healthy cats. *AJVR* 59(4):436–40.

Spears, J.W., et al. 1998. Influence of chromium on glucose metabolism and insulin sensitivity. In *1998 Iams Nutrition Symposium Proceedings.* Vol. 2,

Recent advances in canine and feline nutrition, ed. G.A. Reinhart and D.P. Cary, p. 103. Wilmington Ohio: Orange Frazier Press.

Spiller, R.C. 1994. Pharmacology of dietary fibre. *Pharmac Ther* 62:407–27.

Stauder, G., W. Pollinger, and C. Fruth. 1990. Systemische Enzymtherapie. *Allgemeinmedizin* 19:188–91.

Steinberg, D., G. Kaine, and I. Gedalia. 1996. Antibacterial effect of propolis and honey on oral bacteria. *Am J Dent* 9(6):236–39.

Taboada, J., and D.S. Dimski. 1995. Hepatic encephalopathy: Clinical signs, pathogenesis, and treatment. *Veterinary Clinics of North America* 25(2):357–73.

Takaisi-Kikuni, N.B., and H. Schilcher. 1994. Electron microscopic and microcalorimetric investigations of the possible mechanism of the antibacterial action of a defined propolis provenance. *Planta Medica* 60(3):222–27.

Tarnopolsky, M., and J. Martin. 1999. Creatine monohydrate increases strength in patients with neuromuscular disease. *Neurology* 52(4):854–57.

Twedt, D.C., R.J. Sokol, M.W. Devereaux, and E. Gumprich. 1998. Vitamin E protects against oxidatative damage of bile acids in isolated hepatocytes. *JVIM* 12:215.

Verma, S., M.C. Cam, and J.H. McNeill. 1998. Nutritional factors that can favorably influence the glucose/insulin system: Vanadium. *Journal of the American College of Nutrition* 17(1):11–18.

Weiss, R.C. 1992. Immunologic responses in healthy random source cats fed N,N-dimethylglycine-supplemented diets. *Am J Vet Res* 53(5):829–33.

Welton, A.F., L.D. Tobias, C. Fiedler-Nagy, W. Anderson, W. Hope, K. Meyers, and J.W. Coffey. 1986. Effect of flavonoids on arachidonic acid metabolism. *Prog Clin Biol Res* 213:231–42.

Werbach, M. 1997. *Foundations of nutritional medicine.* Tarzana, California: Third Line Press.

Willard, M.D. 1996. Fructooligosaccharides. In *Proceedings of the American College of Veterinary Internal Medicine, San Antonio, Texas.* Lakewood, Colorado: ACVIM.

Chapter 5

Botanical
Materia Medica

U nless otherwise noted, doses are proportional to weight, that is, the recommended dose for humans should be used to calculate the appropriate dose for an animal by using the proportion of the animal's weight to a human's weight. A standard dosing table derived from veterinary herbalists using this proportional dosing scheme is provided in Table 5.1.

Table 5.1   Dosing suggestions

			Dosage (BID-TID)			
Species/size	Tinctures (drops)	Granules (tsp)	Tablets	Patent pills	Capsules (500 mg)	Loose herbs (tsp)
Canine						
Small	5–10	$1/8$–$1/4$	$1/4$–1	1	$1/3$–$1/2$	$1/2$–$1 1/2$
Medium	10–20	$1/4$–$1/2$	1–2	1–3	$1/2$–1	$1 1/2$–2
Large	20–30	$1/2$–$3/4$	2–3	6–10	1–2	2–3
Giant	30–40	$1/2$–1	3–5	6–10	2–3	3–4
Feline	5–10	$1/8$	$1/4$–$1/2$	2	$1/8$–$1/2$	$1/2$

Source: adapted from Basko 1995 and Silver 1999.
mg = milligram; tsp = teaspoon

Present dosing schemes for herbal medications are fairly arbitrary, and smaller animals may, in fact, metabolize active ingredients more rapidly. Some practitioners prefer dosing herbs by body surface area measurements, similar to the way chemotherapeutic dosages are calculated. This converted dosage is obtained by raising the animal's weight in kilograms to the power 0.666, then dividing by 10. Use this weight, in kilograms, to derive a dose proportional to the labeled human dose for the supplement.

The indications, contraindications, and doses given in the following list are necessarily provisional and experimental.

Aloe vera *(Aloe barbadensis) (Swaim, Riddell, and McGuire 1992; Stuart et al. 1997; Yagi, Yamauchi, and Kuwano 1997; Vazquez et al. 1996)*

Actions

> purgative—increases large intestinal water secretion
>
> immunostimulant (acemannan, a patented extract, contains highest activity)
>
> may stimulate fibroblast growth, modulates wound glycosaminoglycan levels
>
> anti-inflammatory—may inhibit cyclooxygenase

Use

> wound healing
>
> skin or ear inflammation

Contraindications

> none described

Adverse effects

> diarrhea, with oral use of certain forms

Potential interactions

> caution with stool softeners

Dose

> up to 1,500 mg/kg/day of acemannan was administered orally to dogs for 90 days without ill effect

Ashwaganda *(Withania somnifera) (Bone 1996)*

Action

> supports lean body weight gain
>
> anti-inflammatory

Use

> Ayurvedic tonic
>
> anemia
>
> chronic inflammatory conditions
>
> chronic debilitating conditions

NOTE: Question mark indicates research may be reported but is scarce or doubtful in conclusions.

Contraindications
     none described

Adverse effects
     none described

Potential interactions
     none known

Dose
     proportional

Astragalus *(Astragalus membranaceous) (Sinclair 1998; Chu, Wong, and Mavligit 1988)*

Action
     immunostimulant
     classic traditional Chinese tonic

Use
     immune suppressive conditions, recurrent infections
     immune support of certain chemotherapy patients
     chronic debility

Contraindications
     none described

Adverse effects
     none described

Potential interactions
     none known

Dose
     proportional

Bilberry *(Vaccinium myrtilis) (Bertuglia, Malandrino, and Colantuoni 1995; Bravetti 1989; Scharrer and Ober 1981; Bissett 1994)*

Actions
     contains bioflavonoids called anthocyanosides—potent antioxidants
     improves capillary integrity

Use

vasculopathy

retinopathy

cataract

Contraindications

none described

Adverse effects

none described

Potential interactions

none known

Dose

proportional

Black cohosh *(Cimicifuga racemosa) (Lieberman 1998)*

Actions

estrogenlike effects via receptor and nonreceptor mechanisms
suppresses luteinizing hormone

Use

traditionally used for menopausal and menstrual disorders in women
cat owners use as an alternative to hormonal or drug therapy for
inappropriate elimination—probably ineffective

Contraindications

pregnancy

Adverse effects

allergic reactions and GI distress have been reported

Potential interactions

none described

Dose

proportional

Black walnut *(Juglans nigra) (Ahmad, Wahid, and Bukhari 1973)*

Actions

has not been investigated as an anthelmintic though touted as such
may be fungistatic

Use
> very popular among some pet owners as a heartworm preventive and
> intestinal dewormer
> traditional remedy for intestinal parasites

Contraindications
> none described

Adverse effects
> in small animals, reports of toxicity due to a fungal contaminant

Potential interactions
> none known

Dose
> proportional

Boswellia *(Boswellia serrata) (Gupta et al. 1998; Monograph 1998a; Wildfeuer et al. 1998)*

Actions
> anti-inflammatory: boswellic acids are lipoxygenase inhibitors

Use
> osteoarthritis?
> rheumatoid arthritis
> colitis, inflammatory bowel disease
> asthma
> autoimmune disease

Contraindications
> none described

Adverse effects
> Diarrhea, skin inflammation, nausea have been reported in humans

Potential interactions
> caution probably warranted with nonsteroidal anti-inflammatory
> drugs until this herb is better investigated

Dose
> proportional

Calendula *(Calendula officinalis) (Klouchek-Popova et al. 1982; Akihisa et al. 1996; Della Loggia et al. 1994; Zitterl-Eglseer et al. 1997)*

Actions

> anti-inflammatory
> promotes epithelialization

Use

> focal skin irritation
> otitis
> may be used for gastritis and gastric ulcers for the topical effects
> burns

Contraindications

> none described

Adverse effects

> hypersensitivity reactions occasionally reported in people

Potential interactions

> none described

Dose

> topically as needed

Catnip *(Nepeta cataria) (Aydin et al. 1998; Grognet 1990)*

Actions

> psychotropic for cats; mechanism not understood
> nepetalactone, composing 70–99% of the essential oil, has opioid
>   activity

Use

> good for low-calorie cat treats
> good for behavior modification—diversions and rewards?

Contraindications

> use of other psychotropic drugs

Adverse effects

> none reported

Potential interactions

> none described

Dose

as occasional treats, in toys or as loose herb

Cat's claw, Una de gato *(Uncaria tomentosa, U. guianensis)* *(Aquino et al. 1991)*

Actions

unknown; some suggestion of immunostimulatory and anti-inflammatory activities

Use

traditional Amazon remedy for cancer, infections, gastroenteritis, and many other maladies

Contraindications

none described

Adverse effects

none described

Potential interactions

none known

Dose

proportional

Chamomile *(Matricaria recutita, M. chamomilla)* *(Salgueiro et al. 1997; Akihisa et al. 1996; Viola et al. 1995; Safayhi et al. 1994; Merfort et al. 1994; Aertgeerts et al. 1985; Bissett 1994)*

Actions

anxiolytic
antioxidant
anti-inflammatory

Use

skin irritation, hot spots
gingivitis, stomatitis
gastritis, gastric ulcers, enteritis
conjunctivitis (see caution about allergy)
insomnia, anxiety

Contraindications
> none described

Adverse effects
> allergic reactions are reported in humans; caution may be advised in
> animals potentially sensitive to other members of the family
> Compositae, including ragweed.

Potential interactions
> none described

Dose
> proportional

Coleus forskolii *(Coleus forskolii) (Bone 1996)*

Actions
> activates adenylate cyclase
> causes peripheral vasodilation, hypotension
> may increase myocardial contractility
> bronchodilation
> reduces intraocular pressure by reducing aqueous humor production
> suppresses mast cell degranulation

Use
> asthma
> some cases of congestive heart failure, especially dilated
> cardiomyopathy
> hypertension
> glaucoma, topically
> allergy?

Contraindications
> use cautiously in presence of cardiovascular drugs

Adverse effects
> none described

Potential interactions
> concurrent use of drugs with similar activity

Dose
> proportionate

Cranberry *(Vaccinium macrocarpon) (Ahuja, Kaack, and Roberts 1998; Tsukada et al. 1994)*

Actions

bacteriostatic: prevents *E. coli* adherence to bladder mucosa

thought, perhaps erroneously, to acidify urine

Use

prevention of recurrent urinary tract infection

Contraindications

none described

Adverse effects

none described

Potential interactions

none known

Dose

proportional

look for concentrated extracts or powders; doses of cranberry juice are too large to force-feed to animals

Dandelion *(Taraxacum officinale) (Grases et al. 1994; Bissett 1994)*

Actions

mild cholagogue

urinary antiseptic, diuretic

Use

traditional tonic and salad constituent

hepatocellular disease

urinary calculi

Contraindications

cholestatic disease, obstruction of bile duct

Adverse effects

contact dermatitis and allergic reactions in people

Potential interactions

none described

Dose

proportional

Devil's claw *(Harpophogytum procumbens) (Bonnett and Poland 1997; Moussard et al. 1992)*

Actions

suggested as an anti-inflammatory, but evidence suggests that this
effect is minimal or nonexistent
negative chronotrope, antiarrhythmic

Use

osteoarthritis

Contraindications

none described

Adverse effects

none described

Potential interactions

none known

Dose

proportional

Echinacea *(Echinacea purpurea, E. angustifolia) (Melchart et al. 1995; Roesler et al. 1991; Bone 1997)*

Important Note: Echinacea may be an endangered plant, and many herbalists attempt to use alternative immunostimulant plants, such as reishi
mushroom, or use cultivated echinacea as opposed to wild crafted.

Actions

stimulates nonspecific immunity
may have bacteriostatic action by virtue of hyaluronidase inhibitors
anti-inflammatory
evidence in vitro much more promising than in vivo evidence

Use

chronic infections
bacterial infections
traditional remedy for snakebite

Contraindications
>traditional contraindication for use for autoimmune conditions—not investigated

Adverse effects
>rare allergic hypersensitivities reported

Potential interactions
>none described

Dose
>proportional

Eleutherococcus, Siberian ginseng, white ginseng *(Eleutherococcus senticosus, Acanthopanax senticosus) (McRae 1996; Dowling et al. 1996; Bohn, Nebe, and Birr 1987; Yun and Choi 1995)*

Actions
>used traditionally by Russian athletes to improve performance; recent evidence does not substantiate
>traditional cancer preventive—not as effective as panax ginseng
>may enhance immune function
>may ameliorate the effects of radiation and certain toxins

Use
>traditional tonic: many chronic and geriatric disorders characterized by "weakness"

Contraindications
>none described

Adverse effects
>eleuthero is not associated as strongly with adverse effects as is panax

Potential interactions
>may increase digoxin levels with concurrent use

Dose
>proportional

Ephedra, Ma Huang *(Ephedra sinica) (White et al. 1997; Harada and Nishimura 1981)*

Actions

> contains ephedrine and pseudoephedrine, which are
> sympathomimetics

Use

> this drug should be used alone with great caution, if at all; traditional
> uses are always in combination with other herbs
> asthma
> incontinence?

Contraindications

> hypertension, hyperthyroidism, glaucoma, cardiovascular disease

Adverse effects

> may be completely contraindicated in cats, who are said to exhibit
> idiosyncratic reactions frequently

Potential interactions

> MAO inhibitor use, sympathomimetic drugs

Dose

> proportional

Eyebright *(Euphrasia officinalis) (Bissett 1994)*

Actions

> astringent properties of tannin constituents probably account for
> anti-inflammatory action

Use

> conjunctivitis
> keratitis

Contraindications

> none reported

Adverse effects

> because its primary use is as a topical ophthalmic, sterility is a
> concern

Potential interactions
> none described

Dose
> used as a tea compress, or available commercially as several brands of sterile ophthalmic drops—use TID

Garlic *(Allium sativum)* *(Nagourney 1998)*

Actions
> antibacterial, antifungal, antiviral
> peripheral vasodilation
> antithrombotic
> inhibits cholesterol and triglyceride production
> cancer chemopreventive

Use
> chronic infections of various sorts
> cancer preventive, suppresses growth of cancer cells
> lowers blood lipids?
> hypertension?

Contraindications
> none described

Adverse effects
> high doses are likely to cause Heinz body anemia in cats and dogs
> anticoagulant effects may be a concern in animals undergoing surgery

Potential interactions
> none described

Dose
> proportional

Ginger *(Zingiber officinale)* *(Schmid et al. 1994; Aikins and Murphy 1998; Sharma et al. 1997; Sharma, Srivastava, and Gan 1994)*

Actions
> antiemetic
> antioxidant
> lipoxygenase inhibitor

Use

> motion sickness
> nausea
> gastric ulceration
> morning sickness in women
> arthritis

Contraindications

> none described

Adverse effects

> may increase bleeding times

Potential interactions

> none described

Dose

> proportional

Ginkgo *(Ginkgo biloba) (Oken, Storzbach, and Kaye 1998; Itil et al. 1998; Marcilhac et al. 1998; Winter 1998; Chen, Salwinski, and Lee 1997; Kobuchi et al. 1997; White, Scates, and Cooper 1996)*

Actions

> antioxidant
> anticoagulant (antagonizes platelet activating factor)
> improves vascular relaxation via inhibition of nitric oxide
> reduces adrenal peripheral benzodiazepine receptors (altering
>   corticosteroid secretion?)
> monoamine oxidase A and B inhibitors

Use

> senile dementia
> early hyperadrenocorticism
> cardiovascular disease, asthma, circulatory disorders

Contraindications

> coagulopathy, possibly surgery

Adverse effects

> has been associated with coagulation defects

Potential interactions
>   anticoagulant drugs

Dose
>   proportional

Ginseng *See* **Eleutherococcus and Panax**

Goldenseal *(Hydrastis canadensis) (Birdsall and Kelly 1997)*

Important Note: Goldenseal is an endangered plant, and herbalists commonly use alternative plants also containing a main constituent—berberine, such as Oregon grape, Coptis, and Berberis.

Actions (based on berberine)
>   antibacterial, antiamebic, anti-giardia
>   calcium channel agonist?—positive inotrope, antiarrhythmic
>   increases small intestinal transit time

Use
>   congestive heart failure?
>   bacterial diarrhea
>   bacterial infection

Contraindications
>   displaces bilirubin from albumin; not for use in icteric patients

Adverse effects
>   high doses: gi signs, hypotension
>   dogs have been administered 45mg/kg berberine IV without ill effect

Potential interactions
>   none reported

Dose
>   proportional

Grape seed *(Vitis vinifera) (Bagchi et al. 1997; Zafirov et al. 1990)*

Actions
>   pycnogenol—antioxidant effects may be more potent than
>   vitamin C
>   improves capillary integrity

Use

chronic inflammatory conditions, such as autoimmune disorders, infections, etc.

microvascular disease

Contraindications

none described

Adverse effects

none described

Potential interactions

none described

Dose

proportional

Green tea *(Camellia sinensis) (Bushman 1998)*

Actions

catechin and epillocatechin gallate are antioxidants

Use

chemopreventive for several types of cancer

improves lipid profiles in humans

Contraindications

none described

Adverse effects

none described

Potential interactions

none known

Dose

proportional—much of the more promising research is based on epidemiologic evidence from Asian populations ingesting three or more cups of tea daily. Concentrated extracts are available commercially.

Gymnema *(Gymnema sylvestre) (Bone 1996; Chattopadhyay 1998)*

Actions

    may increase insulin production

    may increase insulin sensitivity

Use

    diabetes, as an adjunct to insulin therapy (may help stabilize glucose levels and insulin dose)

Contraindications

    none described

Adverse effects

    none described

Potential interactions

    none described

Dose

    proportional

    hypoglycemic effect is gradual in onset

Gypsywort *(Lycopus europaeus, L. americanus, or L. virginicum)*
(Winterhoff et al. 1994; Auf'mkolk et al. 1984)

Actions

    reduces T3 and T4 levels

    inhibits TSH receptor binding

Use

    suggested for feline hyperthyroidism; if primary mechanism is by inhibiting TSH binding, utility is doubtful

Contraindications

    none described

Adverse effects

    none described

Potential interactions

    none described

Dose

    proportional

Hawthorn *(Crataegus oxycantha)* *(Weihmayr and Ernst 1996; Weikl et al. 1996; Schussler, Holzl, and Fricke 1995)*

Actions

positive inotrope

peripheral vasodilator

may improve coronary blood flow

may act as an ACE inhibitor

antioxidant

Use

dilated cardiomyopathy

congestive heart failure

Contraindications

hypertrophic cardiomyopathy due to positive inotrope action?

Adverse effects

none described

Potential interactions

none described

Dose

proportional

Hops *(Humulus lupulus)* *(Bissett 1994; Duncan, Hare, and Buck 1997)*

Actions

sedative?

Use

anxiety

insomnia

Contraindications

none described

Adverse effects

allergy occasionally reported

malignant hyperthermia reported after ingestion of spent beer hops
  by five dogs (four of which were greyhounds)

Potential interactions
> none described

Dose
> proportional

Horsetail *(Equisetum arvense) (Perez, Laguna, and Walkowski 1985; Bissett 1994)*

Actions
> weak diuretic
> contains bioflavonoids, a high concentration of silicates, and
>> thiaminase

Use
> diuresis
> traditionally used for ascites
> traditional arthritis treatment
> traditional hemostatic (topically and orally)

Contraindications
> none described

Adverse effects
> thiaminase may be a problem in the raw, uncooked herb; tinctures or
>> cooked preparations are recommended
> dermatitis reported rarely

Potential interactions
> none described

Dose
> proportional

Kava kava *(Piper methysticum) (Gleitz et al. 1996; Davies et al. 1992; Jussofie, Schmiz, and Hiemke 1994; Baum, Hill, and Rommelspacher 1998; Seitz et al. 1997)*

Actions
> may modulate multiple neurotransmitter systems including GABA
>> and MAO/dopamine/5-HT
> sedative

anticonvulsant
muscle relaxation
analgesia?

Use

anxiety
intervertebral disk disease
seizures?

Contraindications

none described

Adverse effects

not recommended for long-term use
occasional GI effects have been observed
scaly dermatitis noted in humans after long-term use

Potential interactions

Not for use with other antipsychotics; coma has resulted from
concurrent use with alprazolam

Dose

proportional
use alcohol extract or whole herb (as opposed to teas or decoctions)
for greatest sedative effects

Kelp *(Laminaria sp.; Fucus sp.) (Rasooly, Burek, and Rose 1996)*

Actions

iodine source, as well as other trace minerals
touted as useful in thyroid disease

Use

trace mineral supplement

Contraindications

possibly autoimmune thyroid disease

Adverse effects

iodine may augment autoimmune response against thyroid tissue

Potential interactions
>   none described

Dose
>   proportional

Licorice *(Glycyrrhiza glabra, Glycyrrhiza uralensis) (Duax and Ghosh 1997; Dehpour et al. 1994; Ishii and Fujii 1982; Paolini et al. 1998; Bissett 1994)*

Actions
>   may decrease gastric HCl (hydrochloric acid) and gastrin production
>   anti-inflammatory
>   glycyrrhizin inhibits glucocorticoid clearance
>   choleretic
>   expectorant
>   antiviral?

Use
>   gastritis, gastric ulceration
>   bronchitis

Contraindications
>   none described

Adverse effects
>   many documented cases of hyperaldosteronism from prolonged use,
>   causing hypertension, hyperkalemia, etc.
>   deglycyrrhizinated licorice (DGL) is the safest form, but it may not
>   be as effective

Potential interactions
>   induces cytochrome P-450 dependent activities; may alter
>   metabolism of many other drugs

Dose
>   proportional

Maitake *(Grifola frondosa) (Chang 1996; Nanba 1995)*

Actions
>   beta D-glucan and other polysaccharides stimulate nonspecific
>   immunity

Use
> cancer
> immune suppression, chronic infections

Contraindications
> none described

Adverse effects
> none described

Potential interactions
> none described

Dose
> proportional

Milk thistle *(Silybum marianum) (Thamsborg et al. 1996; Rui 1991; Flora et al. 1998)*

Action
> silymarin, a bioflavonoid complex, is an antioxidant
> protects hepatocytes from toxic insults
> stabilizes hepatocyte membranes by preventing lipid peroxidation
> supports hepatocyte regeneration
> hypocholesterolemic, increases high-density lipoproteins

Use
> especially indicated for toxic insults to the liver
> hepatitis, cholangiohepatitis

Contraindications
> none described

Adverse effects
> rare GI effects, such as diarrhea or nausea, have been reported; these
> should be transient

Potential interactions
> none described

Dose
> proportional

Mullein *(Verbascum thapsus) (Bissett 1994)*

Action

mucilage or saponins may have a demulcent effect

Use

bronchitis, tracheitis
topically, for ear irritation

Contraindications
none described

Adverse effects
none described

Potential interactions
none described

Dose

proportional

Myrrh (*Commiphora molmol* and other *Commiphora* species) *(Bissett 1994)*

Action

not well described

Use

traditional remedy for periodontal infections and inflammation

Contraindications
none described

Adverse effects
allergic contact dermatitis has been reported

Potential interactions
none described

Dose

topically

Neem *(Azadirachta indica) (Guerrini and Kriticos 1998; Zafirov et al. 1990; Talwar et al. 1997; SaiRam et al. 1997; Wolinsky et al. 1996)*

Actions
insect growth regulator
may be antiviral
immunomodulator
abortifacient
inhibits bacterial adhesion to tooth surfaces

Use
parasiticide; especially fleas and mosquitoes
may have use in contraception in the future, as pessary or infusion
periodontal disease

Contraindications
none described

Adverse effects
none reported, though lab animal studies suggest changes in
detoxification enzymes in multiple organs, and at high doses
intravenously, bradyarrhythmias and hypotension

Potential interactions
none described

Dose
topically, as directed by product label

Nettles, Stinging nettle *(Urtica dioica) (Mittman 1990; Hryb et al. 1995; Bissett 1994)*

Actions
stinging hairs contain pro-inflammatory leukotrienes and histamine,
yet the herb is used for its anti-inflammatory effects

Use
allergic rhinitis
benign prostatic hypertrophy
traditional remedy for rheumatoid arthritis

Contraindications
none described

Adverse effects
> none reported except the well-known reaction of skin irritation on contact with fresh nettles

Potential interactions
> none described

Dose
> proportional

Oats *(Avena sativa)*

Action
> unknown

Use
> traditional tranquilizer
> pruritic dermatitis

Contraindications
> none described

Adverse effects
> none described

Potential interactions
> none described

Dose
> proportional
> topically as an infusion to be used as a dip

Panax ginseng (Red ginseng, Korean ginseng) *(Gillis 1997; Sotaniemi, Haapakoski, and Rautio 1995; Bone 1996)*

Actions
> antioxidant
> may enhance nitric oxide synthesis
> hypoglycemic
> may enhance cell differentiation
> may improve erectile dysfunction
> may improve immune function

Use

traditional adaptogen and tonic
traditional performance enhancer
diabetes mellitus
cancer

Contraindications

none described

Adverse effects

insomnia, hypertension, irritability in high doses
not for long-term use

Potential interactions

none described

Dose

proportional

Passionflower *(Passiflora incarnata) (Soulimani et al. 1997; Sopranzi et al. 1990; Bissett 1994)*

Actions

anxiolytic in lab animals

Use

traditional sedative

Contraindications

none described

Adverse effects

none described

Potential interactions

none described

Dose

proportional

Pau d'Arco (*Tabebuia impestignosa* and others) *(Anesini and Perez 1993)*

Actions
> antimicrobial

Use
> bacterial infections
> fungal infections
> yeast infections
> very popular for treatment of cancer—unsupported at this time

Contraindications
> none described

Adverse effects
> none described

Potential interactions
> none described

Dose
> proportional; use whole bark capsules, tablets, or tinctures

Peppermint *(Mentha piperita) (Bissett 1994; Pittler and Ernst 1998; Tate 1997)*

Actions
> antispasmodic?

Use
> irritable bowel syndromes (IBS)
> nausea

Contraindications
> none

Adverse effects
> burning sensations from esophagus to rectum have been reported by
> some people

Potential interactions
> none described

Dose
> use enteric coated capsules for IBS

Phyllanthus *(Phyllanthus niruri, P. amarus) (Calixto et al. 1998; Srividya and Periwal 1995; Santos et al. 1995; Bone 1996)*

Actions

> DNA polymerase inhibitor; may have antiviral activity against hepatitis B and human immunodeficiency virus

Use

> pain control
> antiviral

Contraindications

> none described

Adverse effects

> none described

Potential interactions

> none described

Dose

> proportional

Psyllium *(Plantago ovata) (Plumb 1995)*

Actions

> mucilage swells by absorbing water, inducing peristalsis

Use

> simple constipation
> fiber-responsive GI disease

Contraindications

> obstructive bowel disease

Adverse effects

> increase in fecal volume (and frequency) may be viewed as an adverse effect by the pet owner

Potential interactions

> none described

Dose

as labeled (Vetasyl)

as loose herb, ½–2 tsp SID-BID prn

Red raspberry *(Rubus idaeus)*

Actions

unknown

Use

popular pregnancy support to prevent dystocia—unsupported

traditional remedy for diarrhea

Contraindications

none described

Adverse effects

may rarely cause nausea or loose stool at high doses

Potential interactions

none described

Dose

proportional

opinions differ regarding the best regimen for pregnancy support;

many breeders begin treatment early in pregnancy, whereas others

initiate treatment 2 weeks before parturition

Reishi *(Ganoderma lucidum) (Haak-Frendscho et al. 1993; Park et al. 1997; Wang et al. 1997; van der Hem et al. 1995)*

Actions

immunomodulatory: T-cell mitogen

hepatoprotective; antifibrotic?

Use

cancer

hepatic disease

postsurgical transplantation

Contraindications

none described

Adverse effects
>   rarely, GI effects, bleeding problems, and dizziness have occurred in
>   people using reishi for 3–6 months

Potential interactions
>   none described

Dose
>   proportional

Saw palmetto *(Serenoa repens) (Wilt et al. 1998; Monograph 1998b; Griffiths et al. 1996)*

Actions
>   5-alpha reductase inhibitor—suppresses testosterone formation

Use
>   benign prostatic hypertrophy

Contraindications
>   none described

Adverse effects
>   none described

Potential interactions
>   none described

Dose
>   proportional
>   active constituents are in the lipophilic portion of the extract;
>   therefore, use of alcohol tincture or whole dried herb is preferred
>   to teas

Senna *(Cassia senna, C. angustifolia) (Bissett 1994)*

Actions
>   anthroquinone glycosides increase peristalsis and large intestinal fluid
>   secretion

Use
>   constipation
>   stool softening
>   empty bowel preradiograpy or endoscopy

Contraindications
>   not for use in young puppies and kittens

Adverse effects
>   prolonged use may cause dependence

Potential interactions
>   caution with stool softeners, laxatives

Dose
>   proportional

Slippery elm *(Ulmus fulva)*

Action
>   mucilage may cause bulking of stool

Use
>   very popular traditional remedy for diarrhea of any type
>   traditional remedy for bronchitis, cough

Contraindications
>   intestinal obstruction

Adverse effects
>   none described

Potential interactions
>   none described

Dose
>   proportional

St. John's Wort *(Hypericum perforatum) (Linde et al. 1996; Upton 1997)*

Actions
>   antidepressant; mechanisms may include serotonin reuptake
>   inhibition, MAO inhibition, GABA binding
>   antiviral

Use
>   depression, anxiety
>   retroviral and other viral infection
>   wound healing

Contraindications
> none described

Adverse effects
> photosensitivity

Potential interactions
> not for use with other mood-altering drugs

Dose
> proportional
> use at least 6–8 weeks

Tea tree *(Melaleuca alternifolia) (Concha, Moore, and Holloway 1998; Bischoff and Guale 1998; Hammer, Carson, and Riley 1996)*

Actions
> antifungal
> antibacterial

Use
> focal dermatophytosis

Contraindications
> not for use in cats; anecdotal evidence suggests that some small-breed
> dogs are sensitive to undiluted essential oil as well

Adverse effects
> patch test first, because some animals and people have shown
> sensitivities

Potential interactions
> none described

Dose
> topical, may dilute 50% with vegetable oil

Turmeric *(Curcuma longa) (Sreejayan and Rao 1996; Kuo and Huang 1996; Srivastava, Bordia, and Verma 1995; Sidhu et al. 1998; Deshpande et al. 1998; Huang, Newmark, and Frenkel 1997)*

Actions
> inhibits carcinogenesis
> lipoxygenase inhibitor

antioxidant
hepatoprotective
enhances wound healing
prevents platelet aggregation

Use

hepatitis
cancer
many inflammatory conditions

Contraindications

none described

Adverse effects

none described

Potential interactions

none described

Dose

proportional

Uva ursi *(Arctostaphylos uva-ursi) (Bissett 1994)*

Actions

bacteriostatic in alkaline urine

Use

UTI

Contraindications

none described
do not use long term

Adverse effects

nausea is occasionally reported in humans

Potential interactions

do not use with urinary acidifiers

Dose

proportional

Valerian *(Valeriana officinalis) (Andreatini and Leite 1994; Schulz, Stolz, and Muller 1994)*

Actions
> sedative—may be GABA-ergic

Use
> insomnia
> anxiety

Contraindications
> none described

Adverse effects
> none described

Potential interactions
> do not use concurrently with barbiturates or benzodiazepines

Dose
> proportional

Venus fly trap *(Dionaea muscipula) (Carnivora) (Kreher et al. 1988; Todorov and Ilarionova 1996)*

Important Note: This is an endangered plant in its native habitat; be aware of sources.

Actions
> antiproliferative?
> immunostimulant

Use
> cancer

Contraindications
> none described

Adverse effects
> none described

Potential interactions
> none described

Dose

> 1 cc SQ for animals under 50 lbs
> 2 cc SQ for animals over 50 lbs
> administer 5 days on, 2 days off

White willow *(Salix alba) (Bissett 1994)*

Actions

> contains salicin, a cyclooxygenase inhibitor (from which
> acetylsalicylic acid was derived)

Use

> used rarely in veterinary medicine
> fever
> rheumatoid arthritis, perhaps osteoarthritis

Contraindications

> none described

Adverse effects

> nausea, diarrhea, gastric ulceration

Potential interactions

> caution is advised with nonsteroidal anti-inflammatory drugs

Dose

> proportional

Wild yam *(Dioscorea villosa, D. floribunda, D. composita)* *(Weiss 1994)*

Notes: industrial source for synthetic steroid synthesis

Actions

> steroidal saponins (e.g., diosgenin) are probably not converted to
> steroid in vivo, and the extent of their native steroidlike activity
> has yet to be determined

Use

> inflammatory bowel disease?
> arthritis?

Contraindications
>   none described

Adverse effects
>   occasional nausea

Potential interactions
>   none described

Dose
>   proportional

Witch hazel *(Hamamelis virginiana) (Bissett 1994)*

Actions
>   tannins are astringent

Use
>   mild focal skin inflammation, "hot spots"

Contraindications
>   OTC forms not for internal use; tea made from bark and leaves is
>   apparently nontoxic

Adverse effects
>   none described

Potential interactions
>   none described

Dose
>   topically

Yucca *(Yucca schidigera)*

Actions
>   Yucca saponins are commonly (and probably mistakenly) believed to
>   have corticosteroidlike activity

Use
>   Osteoarthritis?
>   yucca is probably more useful as a natural soaplike agent

Contraindications
    none described

Adverse effects
    none described

Potential interactions
    none described

Dose
    proportional

Herbs that are potentially toxic even at recommended dosages

    Chaparral
    Comfrey
    Pennyroyal
    Garlic
    Tea tree
    Ma huang/ephedra

References

Aertgeerts, P., M. Albring, F. Klaschka, T. Nasemann, R. Patzelt-Wenczler, K. Rauhut, and B. Weigl. 1985. Comparative testing of Kamillosan cream and steroidal (0.25% hydrocortisone, 0.75% fluocortin butyl ester) and non-steroidal (5% bufexamac) dermatologic agents in maintenance therapy of eczematous diseases. *Z Hautkr* 60(3):270–77.

Ahmad, S., M.A. Wahid, and A.Q. Bukhari. 1973. Fungistatic action of Juglans. *Antimicrob Agents Chemother* 3(3):436–38.

Ahuja, S., B. Kaack, and J. Roberts. 1998. Loss of fimbrial adhesion with the addition of *Vaccinum macrocarpon* to the growth medium of P-fimbriated *Escherichia coli. J Urol* 159(2):559–62.

Aikins Murphy, P. 1998. Alternative therapies for nausea and vomiting of pregnancy. *Obstet Gynecol* 91(1):149–55.

Akihisa, T., K. Yasukawa, H. Oinuma, Y. Kasahara, S. Yamanouchi, M. Takido, K. Kumaki, and T. Tamura. 1996. Triterpene alcohols from the flowers of compositae and their anti-inflammatory effects. *Phytochemistry* 43(6):1255–60.

Andreatini, R., and J.R. Leite. 1994. Effect of valepotriates on the behavior of rats in the elevated plus-maze during diazepam withdrawal. *Eur J Pharmacol* 260(2–3):233–35.

Anesini, C., and C. Perez. 1993. Screening of plants used in Argentine folk medicine for antimicrobial activity. *J Ethnopharmacol* 39(2):119–28.

Aquino, R., V. De Feo, F. De Simone, C. Pizza, and G. Cirino. 1991. Plant metabolites: New compounds and anti-inflammatory activity of Uncaria tomentosa. *J Nat Prod* 54(2):453–59.

Auf'mkolk, M., J.C. Ingbar, S.M. Amir, H. Winterhoff, H. Sourgens, R.D. Hesch, and S.H. Ingbar. 1984. Inhibition by certain plant extracts of the binding and adenylate cyclase stimulatory effect of bovine thyrotropin in human thyroid membranes. *Endocrinology* 115(2):527–34.

Aydin, S., R. Beis, Y. Ozturk, K. Husnu, and C. Baser. 1998. Nepetalactone: A new opioid analgesic from Nepeta caesarea Boiss. *J Pharm Pharmacol* 50(7):813–17.

Bagchi, D., A. Garg, R.L. Krohn, M. Bagchi, M.X. Tran, and S.J. Stohs. 1997. Oxygen free radical scavenging abilities of vitamins C and E, and a grape seed proanthocyanidin extract in vitro. *Res Commun Mol Pathol Pharmacol* 95(2):179–89.

Basko, I. 1995. Over-the-Counter Herbal Pet Supplements: Fact or Fiction? In *Proceedings of the 1995 Annual Conference of the AHVMA; Snowmass, Colorado*, p. 137. Bel Air, Maryland: AHVMA.

Baum, S.S., R. Hill, and H. Rommelspacher. 1998. Effect of kava extract and individual kavapyrones on neurotransmitter levels in the nucleus accumbens of rats. *Prog Neuropsychopharmacol Biol Psychiatry* 22(7):1105–20.

Bertuglia, S., S. Malandrino, and A. Colantuoni. 1995. Effect of *Vaccinium myrtillus* anthocyanosides on ischaemia reperfusion injury in hamster cheek pouch microcirculation. *Pharmacol Res* 31(3–4):183–87.

Birdsall, T.C., and G.S. Kelly. 1997. Berberine: Therapeutic potential of an alkaloid found in several medicinal plants. *Alternative Medicine Review* 2(2):94–103.

Bischoff, K., and F. Guale. 1998. Australian tea tree *(Melaleuca alternifolia)* oil poisoning in three purebred cats. *J Vet Diagn Invest* 10(2):208–10.

Bissett, N. 1994. *Herbal drugs and phytopharmaceuticals: A handbook for practice on a scientific basis*. Boca Raton, Florida: CRC Press.

Bohn, B., C.T. Nebe, and C. Birr. 1987. Flow-cytometric studies with *Eleutherococcus senticosus* extract as an immunomodulatory agent. *Arzneimittelforschung* 37(10):1193–96.

Bone, K. 1996. *Clinical applications of Ayurvedic and Chinese herbs: Monographs for the western herbal practitioner*. Warwick, Queensland, Australia: Phytotherapy Press.

Bone, K. 1997. Echinacea: What makes it work? *Alternative Medicine Review* 2(2):87–93.

Bonnett, B., and C. Poland. 1997. Preliminary results of a randomized double-blind, multicenter, controlled clinical trial of two herbal therapies, acetylsalicylic acid and placebo for osteoarthritis in dogs. In *Proceedings of the 1997 Annual Conference of the AHVMA; Burlington, Vermont*, p. 143. Bel Air, Maryland: AHVMA.

Bravetti, G. 1989. Preventive medical treatment of senile cataract with vitamin E and anthocyanosides: Clinical evaluation. *Ann Ottalmol Clin Ocul* 115:109.

Bushman, J.L. 1998. Green tea and cancer in humans: A review of the literature. *Nutrition and Cancer* 31(3):151–59.

Calixto, J.B., A.R. Santos, V. Cechinel Filho, and R.A. Yunes. 1998. A review of the plants of the genus *Phyllanthus*: Their chemistry, pharmacology, and therapeutic potential. *Med Res Rev* 18(4):225–58.

Chang, R. 1996. Functional properties of edible mushrooms. *Nutr Rev* 54(11 Pt 2):S91–93.

Chattopadhyay, R.R. 1998. Possible mechanism of antihyperglycemic effect of *Gymnema sylvestre* leaf extract, part I. *Gen Pharmacol* 31(3):495–96.

Chen, X., S. Salwinski, and T.J. Lee. 1997. Extracts of *Ginkgo biloba* and ginsenosides exert cerebral vasorelaxation via a nitric oxide pathway. *Clin Exp Pharmacol Physiol* 24:958–59.

Chu, D.T., W.L. Wong, and G.M. Mavligit. 1988. Immunotherapy with Chinese medicinal herbs I: Immune restoration of local xenogenic graft-versus-host reaction in cancer patients by fractioned *Astragalus membranaceus* in vitro. *J Clin Lab Immunol* 25:119–23.

Concha, J.M., L.S. Moore, and W.J. Holloway. 1998. Antifungal activity of *Melaleuca alternifolia* (tea-tree) oil against various pathogenic organisms. *J Am Podiatr Med Assoc* 88(10):489–92.

Davies, L.P., C.A. Drew, P. Duffield, G.A. Johnston, and D.D. Jamieson. 1992. Kava pyrones and resin: Studies on GABAA, GABAB and benzodiazepine binding sites in rodent brain. *Pharmacol Toxicol* 71(2):120–26.

Dehpour, A.R., M.E. Zolfaghari, T. Samadian, and Y. Vahedi. 1994. The protective effect of liquorice components and their derivatives against gastric ulcer induced by aspirin in rats. *J Pharm Pharmacol* 46(2):148–49.

Della Loggia, R., A. Tubaro, S. Sosa, H. Becker, S. Saar, and O. Isaac. 1994. The role of triterpenoids in the anti-inflammatory activity of *Calendula officinalis* flowers. *Planta Med* 60:516–20.

Deshpande, U.R., S.G. Gadre, A.S. Raste, D. Pillai, S.V. Bhide, and A.M. Samuel. 1998. Protective effect of turmeric *(Curcuma longa L.)* extract on carbon tetrachloride–induced liver damage in rats. *Indian J Exp Biol* 36(6):573–77.

Dowling, E.A., D.R. Redondo, J.D. Branch, S. Jones, G. McNabb, and M.H. Williams. 1996. Effect of *Eleutherococcus senticosus* on submaximal and maximal exercise performance. *Med Sci Sports Exerc* 28(4):482–89.

Duax, W.L., and D. Ghosh. 1997. Structure and function of steroid dehydrogenases involved inhypertension, fertility, and cancer. *Steroids* 62(1):95–100.

Duncan, K.L., W.R. Hare, and W.B. Buck. 1997. Malignant hyperthermia-like reaction secondary to ingestion of hops in five dogs. *J Am Vet Med Assoc* 210(1):51–54.

Flora, K., M. Hahn, H. Rosen, and K. Benner. 1998. Milk thistle *(Silybum marianum)* for the therapy of liver disease. *Am J Gastroenterol* 93(2):139–43.

Gaby, A.R. 1996. *Ginkgo biloba* extract: A review. *Alternative Medicine Review* 1(4):236–42.

Gillis, C.N. 1997. Panax ginseng pharmacology: A nitric oxide link? *Biochem Pharmacol* 54(1):1–8.

Gleitz, J., J. Friese, A. Beile, A. Ameri, and T. Peters. 1996. Anticonvulsive action of ±-kavain estimated from its properties on stimulated synaptosomes and Na+ channel receptor sites. *Eur J Pharmacol* 315(1):89–97.

Grases, F., G. Melero, A. Costa-Bauza, R. Prieto, and J.G. March. 1994. Urolithiasis and phytotherapy. *Int Urol Nephrol* 26(5):507–11.

Griffiths, K., H. Adlercreutz, P. Boyle, L. Denis, R.I. Nicholson, and M.S. Morton. 1996. *Nutrition and cancer.* Oxford, England: Isis Medical Media.

Grognet, J. 1990. Catnip: Its uses and effects, past and present. *Can Vet J* 31(6):455–56.

Guerrini, V.H., and C.M. Kriticos. 1998. Effects of azadirachtin on *Ctenocephalides felis* in the dog and the cat. *Vet Parasitol* 74(2–4):289–97.

Gupta, I., V. Gupta, A. Parihar, S. Gupta, R. Ludtke, H. Safayhi, and H.P.T. Ammon. 1998. Effects of *Boswellia serrata* gum resin in patients with bronchial asthma: Results of a double-blind, placebo-controlled, 6-week clinical study. *Eur J Med Res* 3(11):511–14.

Haak-Frendscho, M., K. Kino, T. Sone, and P. Jardieu. 1993. Ling Zhi-8: A novel T cell mitogen induces cytokine production and upregulation of ICAM-1 expression. *Cell Immunol* 150(1):101–13.

Hammer, K.A., C.F. Carson, T.V. Riley. 1996. Susceptibility of transient and commensal skin flora to the essential oil of *Melaleuca alternifolia* (tea tree oil). *Am J Infect Control* 24(3):186–89.

Harada, M., and M. Nishimura. 1981. Contribution of alkaloid fraction to pressor and hyperglycemic effect of crude *Ephedra* extract in dogs. *J Pharmacobiodyn* 4(9):691–99.

Hryb, D.J., M.S. Khan, N.A. Romas, and W. Rosner. 1995. The effect of extracts of the roots of the stinging nettle *(Urtica dioica)* on the interaction of SHBG with its receptor on human prostatic membranes. *Planta Med* 61(1):31–2.

Huang, M.T., H.L. Newmark, and K. Frenkel. 1997. Inhibitory effects of curcumin on tumorigenesis in mice. *J Cell Biochem Suppl* 27:26–34.

Ishii, Y., and Y. Fujii. 1982. Effects of FM100, a fraction of licorice root, on serum gastrin concentrations in rats and dogs. *Jpn J Pharmacol* 32(1):23–27.

Itil, T.M., E. Eralp, I. Ahmed, A. Kunitz, and K.Z. Itil. 1998. The pharmacological effects of *Ginkgo biloba*, a plant extract, on the brain of dementia patients in comparison with tacrine. *Psychopharmacol Bull* 34(3):391–97.

Jahodar, L., I. Leifertova, and M. Lisa. 1978. Investigation of iridoid substances in *Arctostaphylos uva-ursi*. *Pharmazie* 33(8):536–37.

Jussofie, A., A. Schmiz, and C. Hiemke. 1994. Kavapyrone enriched extract from *Piper methysticum* as modulator of the GABA binding site in different regions of rat brain. *Psychopharmacology (Berl)* 116(4):469–74.

Klouchek-Popova, E., A. Popov, N. Pavlova, and S.L. Krusteva. 1982. Influence of the physiological regeneration and epithelialization using fractions isolated from *Calendula officinalis*. *Acta Physiol Pharmacol Bulg* 8(4):63–67.

Kobuchi, H., M.T. Droy-Lefaix, Y. Christen, and L. Packer. 1997. *Ginkgo biloba* extract (Egb 761): Inhibitory effect on nitric oxide production in the macrophage cell line RAW 264.7. *Biochem Pharmacol* 53:897–903.

Kreher, B.A., A. Neszmelyi, K. Polos, and H. Wagner. 1988. Structure elucidation of plumbagin-analogues from *Dionaea muscipula* and their immunomodulating activities in vitro and in vivo. *Molecular Recognition Intern. Symposium. Sopron, Hungary, August 24–27, 1988.* Budapest: Hungarian Academy of Sciences.

Kuo, M.L., and T.S. Huang. 1996. Curcumin, an antioxidant and anti-tumor promoter, induces apoptosis in human leukemia cells. *Biochim Biophys Acta* 1317(2):95–100.

Lieberman S. 1998. A review of the effectiveness of *Cimicifuga racemosa* (black cohosh) for the symptoms of menopause. *J Womens Health* 7(5):525–29.

Linde, K., G. Ramirez, C.D. Mulrow, A. Pauls, W. Weidenhammer, and D. Melchart. 1996. St. John's Wort for depression—An overview and meta-analysis of randomised clinical trials. *BMJ* 313:253–58.

Marcilhac, A., N. Dakine, N. Bourhim, V. Guillaume, M. Grino, K. Drieu, and C. Oliver. 1998. Effect of chronic administration of *Ginkgo biloba* extract or Ginkgolide on the hypothalamic-pituitary-adrenal axis in the rat. *Life Sci* 62(25):2329–40.

McRae, S. 1996. Elevated serum digoxin levels in a patient taking digoxin and Siberian ginseng. *CMAJ* 155(3):293–95.

Melchart, D., K. Linde, F. Worku, L. Sarkady, M. Holzmann, K. Jurcic, and H. Wagner. 1995. Results of five randomized studies on the immunomodulatory activity of preparations of *Echinacea. J Altern Complement Med* 1(2):145–60.

Merfort, I., J. Heilmann, U. Hagedorn-Leweke, and B.C. Lippold. 1994. In vivo skin penetration studies of camomile flavones. *Pharmazie* 49(7):509–11.

Mittman, P. 1990. Randomized, double-blind study of freeze-dried *Urtica dioica* in the treatment of allergic rhinitis. *Planta Med* 56(1):44–47.

Monograph 1998a. *Boswellia serrata. Altern Med Rev* 3(4):306–7.

Monograph 1998b. *Serenoa repens. Altern Med Rev* 3(3):227–29.

Moussard, C., D. Alber, M.M. Toubin, N. Thevenon, and J.C. Henry. 1992. A drug used in traditional medicine, harpagophytum procumbens: No evidence for NSAID-like effect on whole blood eicosanoid production in human. *Prostaglandins Leukot Essent Fatty Acids* 46(4):283–86.

Nagourney, R.A. 1998. Garlic: Medicinal food or nutritious medicine? *Journal of Medicinal Food* 1(1):13–28.

Nanba, H. 1995. Activity of Maitake D-fraction to inhibit carcinogenesis and metastasis. *Ann N Y Acad Sci.* 768:243–45.

Oken, B.S., D.M. Storzbach, and J.A. Kaye. 1998. The efficacy of *Ginkgo biloba* on cognitive function in Alzheimer disease. *Arch Neurol* 55(11):1409–15.

Paolini, M., L. Pozzetti, A. Sapone, and G. Cantelli-Forti. 1998. Effect of licorice and glycyrrhizin on murine liver CYP-dependent monooxygenases. *Life Sci* 62(6):571–82.

Park, E.J., G. Ko, J. Kim, and D.H. Sohn. 1997. Antifibrotic effects of a polysaccharide extracted from *Ganoderma lucidum*, glycyrrhizin, and pentoxifylline in rats with cirrhosis induced by biliary obstruction. *Biol Pharm Bull* 20(4):417–20.

Perez Gutierrez, R.M., G.Y. Laguna, and A. Walkowski. 1985. Diuretic activity of Mexican equisetum. *J Ethnopharmacol* 14(2–3):269–72.

Pittler, M.H., and E. Ernst. 1998. Peppermint oil for irritable bowel syndrome: A critical review and metaanalysis. *Am J Gastroenterol* 93(7):1131–35.

Plumb, D.C. 1995. *Veterinary drug handbook.* 2nd ed. Ames: Iowa State University Press.

Rasooly, L., C.L. Burek, and N.R. Rose. 1996. Iodine-induced autoimmune thyroiditis in NOD-H-2h4 mice. *Clin Immunol Immunopathol* 81(3):287–92.

Roesler, J., C. Steinmuller, A. Kiderlen, A. Emmendorffer, H. Wagner, and M.L. Lohmann-Matthes. 1991. Application of purified polysaccharides from cell cultures of the plant *Echinacea purpurea* to mice mediates protection against systemic infections with *Listeria monocytogenes* and *Candida albicans*. *Int J Immunopharmacol* 13(1):27–37.

Rui, Y.C. 1991. Advances in pharmacological studies of silymarin. *Mem Inst Oswaldo Cruz* 86(Suppl 2):79–85.

Safayhi, H., J. Sabieraj, E.R. Sailer, and H.P. Ammon. 1994. Chamazulene: An antioxidant-type inhibitor of leukotriene B4 formation. *Planta Med* 60(5):410–13.

SaiRam, M., S.K. Sharma, G. Ilavazhagan, D. Kumar, and W. Selvamurthy. 1997. Immunomodulatory effects of NIM-76, a volatile fraction from neem oil. *J Ethnopharmacol* 55(2):133–39.

Salgueiro, J.B., P. Ardenghi, M. Dias, M.B. Ferreira, I. Izquierdo, and J.H. Medina. 1997. Anxiolytic natural and synthetic flavonoid ligands of the central benzodiazepine receptor have no effect on memory tasks in rats. *Pharmacol Biochem Behav* 58(4):887–91.

Santos, A.R., V.C. Filho, R.A. Yunes, and J.B. Calixto. 1995. Analysis of the mechanisms underlying the antinociceptive effect of the extracts of plants from the genus *Phyllanthus*. *Gen Pharmacol* 26(7):1499–1506.

Scharrer, A., and M. Ober. 1981. Anthocyanosides in the treatment of retinopathies. *Klin Monastbl Aukenheilkd* 178:386–89.

Schmid, R., T. Schick, R. Steffen, A. Tschopp, and T. Wilk. 1994. Comparison of seven commonly used agents for prophylaxis of seasickness. *J Travel Med* 1(4):203–6.

Schulz, H., C. Stolz, and J. Muller. 1994. The effect of valerian extract on sleep polygraphy in poor sleepers: A pilot study. *Pharmacopsychiatry* 27(4):147–51.

Schussler, M., J. Holzl, and U. Fricke. 1995. Myocardial effects of flavonoids from *Crataegus* species. *Arzneimittel-Forschung* 45(8):842–45.

Seitz, U., A. Ameri, H. Pelzer, J. Gleitz, and T. Peters. 1997. Relaxation of evoked contractile activity of isolated guinea-pig ileum by ±-kavain. *Planta Med* 63(4):303–6.

Sharma, S.S., V. Kochupillai, S.K. Gupta, S.D. Seth, and Y.K. Gupta. 1997. Antiemetic efficacy of ginger *(Zingiber officinale)* against cisplatin-induced emesis in dogs. *J Ethnopharmacol* 57(2):93–96.

Sharma, J.N., K.C. Srivastava, and E.K. Gan. 1994. Suppressive effects of eugenol and ginger oil on arthritic rats. *Pharmacology* 49(5):314–18.

Sidhu, G.S., A.K. Singh, D. Thaloor, K.K. Banaudha, G.K. Patnaik, R.C. Srimal, and R.K. Maheshwari. 1998. Enhancement of wound healing by curcumin in animals. *Wound Repair Regen* 6(2):167–77.

Silver, R. 1999. Practical Therapeutics of Natural Remedies. In *Proceedings of the 60th Annual Conference for Veterinarians, Colorado State University College of Veterinary Medicine and Biomedical Science*, pp. 199–209. Fort Collins, Colorado.

Sinclair, S. 1998. Chinese herbs: A clinical review of astragalus, ligusticum and schizandrae. *Altern Med Rev* 3(5):338–44.

Sopranzi, N., G. De Feo, G. Mazzanti, and L. Tolu. 1990. Biological and electroencephalographic parameters in rats in relation to *Passiflora incarnata* L. *Clin Ter* 132(5):329–33.

Sotaniemi, E.A., E. Haapakoski, and A. Rautio. 1995. Ginseng therapy in non-insulin-dependent diabetic patients. *Diabetes Care* 18(10):1373–75.

Soulimani, R., C. Younos, S. Jarmouni, D. Bousta, R. Misslin, and F. Mortier. 1997. Behavioural effects of *Passiflora incarnata* L. and its indole alkaloid and flavonoid derivatives and maltol in the mouse. *J Ethnopharmacol* 57(1):11–20.

Sreejayan, N., and M.N. Rao. 1996. Free radical scavenging activity of curcuminoids. *Arzneimeittel-Forschung* 46(2):169–71.

Srivastava, K.C., A. Bordia, and S.K. Verma. 1995. Curcumin, a major component of food spice turmeric *(Curcuma longa)* inhibits aggregation and alterns eicosanoid metabolism in human blood platelets. *Prostaglandins Leukot Essent Fatty Acids* 52(4):223–27.

Srividya, N., and S. Periwal. 1995. Diuretic, hypotensive and hypoglycaemic effect of *Phyllanthus amarus*. *Indian J Exp Biol* 33(11):861–64.

Stuart, R.W., D.L. Lefkowitz, J.A. Lincoln, K. Howard, M.P. Gelderman, and S.S. Lefkowitz. 1997. Upregulation of phagocytosis and candidicidal activity of macrophages exposed to the immunostimulant acemannan. *Int J Immunopharmacol* 19(2):75–82.

Swaim, S.F., K. Riddell, and J. McGuire. 1992. Effects of topical medications on the healing of open pad wounds in dogs. *J Am Anim Hosp Assoc* 28(6):499–502.

Talwar, G.P., S. Shah, S. Mukherjee, and R. Chabra. 1997. Induced termination of pregnancy by purified extracts of *Azadirachta indica* (neem): Mechanisms involved. *Am J Reprod Immunol* 37(6):485–91.

Tate, S. 1997. Peppermint oil: A treatment for postoperative nausea. *J Adv Nurs* 26(3):543–49.

Thamsborg, S.M., R.J. Jorgensen, E. Brummerstedt, and J. Bjerregard. 1996. Putative effect of silymarin on sawfly *(Arge pullata)*–induced hepatotoxicosis in sheep. *Vet Hum Toxicol* 38(2):89–91.

Todorov, D.K., and M.V. Ilarionova. 1996. Antitumor activity of the *Dionaea muscipula* E. preparation Carnivora new in vitro and in vivo on several animal and human tumors, sensitive and resistant to antitumor drugs. Nordhalben, Germany: Carnivora-Forschungs-Gmbh.

Tsukada, K., K. Tokunaga, T. Iwama, Y. Mishima, K. Tazawa, and M. Fujimaki. 1994. Cranberry juice and its impact on peri-stomal skin conditions for urostomy patients. *Ostomy Wound Manage* 40(9):60–62, 64, 66–68.

Upton, R., ed. 1997. St. John's Wort *(Hypericum perforatum):* Quality control, analytical and therapeutic monograph. Santa Cruz, California: American Herbal Pharmacopeia.

van der Hem, L.G., J.A. van der Vliet, C.F. Bocken, K. Kino, A.J. Hoitsma, and W.J. Tax. 1995. Ling Zhi-8: Studies of a new immunomodulating agent. *Transplantation* 60(5):438–43.

Vazquez, B., G. Avila, D. Segura, and B. Escalante. 1996. Antiinflammatory activity of extracts from aloe vera gel. *J Ethnopharmacol* 55(1):69–75.

Viola, H., C. Wasowski, M. Levi de Stein, C. Wolfman, R. Silveira, F. Dajas, J.H. Medina, and A.C. Paladini. 1995. Apigenin, a component of *Matricaria recutita* flowers, is a central benzodiazepine receptors-ligand with anxiolytic effects. *Planta Med* 61(3):213–16.

Wang, S.Y., M.L. Hsu, T.C. Hsu, C.H. Tzeng, S.S. Lee, M.S. Shiao, and C.K. Ho. 1997. The anti-tumor effect of Ganoderma lucidum is mediated by cytokines released from activated macrophages and T lymphocytes. *Int J Cancer* 70(6):699–705.

Weihmayr, T., and E. Ernst. 1996. Therapeutic effectiveness of *Crataegus. Fortschr Med* 114(1–2):27–29.

Weikl, A., K.D. Assmus, A. Neukum-Schmidt, J. Schmitz, G. Zapfe, H.S. Noh, and J. Siegrist. 1996. Crataegus Special Extract WS 1442: Assessment of objective effectiveness in patients with heart failure. *Fortschr Med* 114(24):291–96.

Weiss, R. 1994. *Herbal medicine.* Beaconsfield, England: Beaconsfield Publishers Ltd.

White, H.L., P.W. Scates, and B.R. Cooper. 1996. Extracts of *Ginkgo biloba* leaves inhibit monoamine oxidase. *Life Sci* 58:1315–21.

White, L.M., S.F. Gardner, B.J. Gurley, M.A. Marx, P.L. Wang, and M. Estes. 1997. Pharmacokinetics and cardiovascular effects of ma-huang *(Ephedra sinica)* in normotensive adults. *J Clin Pharmacol* 37(2):116–22.

Wildfeuer, A., I.S. Neu, H. Safayhi, G. Metzger, M. Wehrmann, U. Vogel, and H.P. Ammon. 1998. Effects of boswellic acids extracted from a herbal medicine on the biosynthesis of leukotrienes and the course of experimental autoimmune encephalomyelitis. *Arzneimittelforschung* 48(6):668–74.

Wilt, T.J., A. Ishani, G. Stark, R. MacDonald, J. Lau, and C. Mulrow. 1998. Saw palmetto extracts for treatment of benign prostatic hyperplasia. *JAMA* 280:1604–9.

Winter, J.C. 1998. The effects of an extract of *Ginkgo biloba*, EGb 761, on cognitive behavior and longevity in the rat. *Physiol Behav* 63(3):425–33.

Winterhoff, H., H.G. Gumbinger, U. Vahlensieck, F.H. Kemper, H. Schmitz, and B. Behnke. 1994. Endocrine effects of *Lycopus europaeus* L. following oral application. *Arzneimittelforschung* 44(1):41–45.

Wolinsky, L.E., S. Mania, S. Nachnani, and S. Ling 1996. The inhibiting effect of aqueous *Azadirachta indica* (neem) extract upon bacterial properties influencing in vitro plaque formation. *J Dent Res* 75(2):816–22.

Yagi, T., K. Yamauchi, and S. Kuwano. 1997. The synergistic purgative action of aloe-emodin anthrone and rhein anthrone in mice: Synergism in large intestinal propulsion and water secretion. *J Pharm Pharmacol* 49(1):22–25.

Yun, T.K., and S.Y. Choi. 1995. Preventive effect of ginseng intake against various human cancers: A case control study of 1987 pairs. *Cancer Epidemiology, Biomarkes and Prevention* 4:401–8.

Zafirov, D., G. Bredy-Dobreva, V. Litchev, and M. Papasova. 1990. Antiexudative and capillaritonic effects of procyanidines isolated from grape seeds *(V. vinifera)*. *Acta Physiol Pharmacol Bulg* 16(3):50–54.

Zeitlin, L., K.J. Whaley, T.A. Hegarty, T.R. Moench, and R.A. Cone. 1997. Tests of vaginal microbicides in the mouse genital herpes model. *Contraception* 56(5):329–35.

Zitterl-Eglseer, K., S. Sosa, J. Jurenitsch, M. Schubert-Zsilavecz, R. Della Loggia, A. Tubaro, M. Bertoldi, and C. Franz. 1997. Anti-oedematous activities of the main triternoil esters of marigold (*Calendula officinalis* L). *J Ethnopharmacol* 57:139–44.

Training and Related Organizations

Training and Certification

Academy of Veterinary Homeopathy

751 NE 168th Street

North Miami Beach, FL 33162

Phone: 305-652-1590

Fax: 305-653-7244

Fax on Demand: 305-653-3337

E-mail: avh@naturalholistic.com

Website: http//www.acadvethom.org

Offers four-module, 1-year course in veterinary
classical homeopathy.

American Academy of Veterinary Acupuncture

P.O. Box 419

Hygiene, CO 80433-0419

Phone/fax: 303-772-6726

E-mail: AAVAoffice@aol.com

Sponsors advanced seminars for veterinarians with basic
training in acupuncture and traditional Chinese
medicine.

American Holistic Veterinary Medical Association

2214 Old Emmorton Road

Bel Air, MD 21014

Phone: 410-569-0795

Fax: 410-569-2346

E-mail: AHVMA@compuserve.com

Not a training organization per se but has an excellent annual
conference and a journal related to all alternative or holistic therapies.

American Veterinary Chiropractic Association

623 Main

Hillsdale, IL 61257

Phone: 309-658-2920

Fax: 309-658-2622

Offers five-module, 2-year course in veterinary chiropractic leading to
certification.

Chi Institute of Chinese Medicine

9791 NW 160th Street

Reddick, FL 32686

Phone: 352-591-3165

Fax: 352-591-0988

E-mail: HolisticEq@aol.com

Offers 120 hours of instruction in four modules, which covers
veterinary acupuncture and qualifies veterinarians to take the IVAS
certification exam, and a 120-hour course on traditional Chinese
herbal medicine.

International Veterinary Acupuncture Society

P.O. Box 1478

Longmont, CO 80502

Phone: 303-682-1167

Fax: 303-682-1168

E-mail: IVASOffice@aol.com

Acupuncture course is approximately 120 hours of training (four modules
over 6 months), which qualifies veterinarians to take the certification
exam.

Chinese herbal medicine course is offered only to IVAS acupuncture-certified veterinarians. It is a three-year, six-module course covering aspects of traditional Chinese herbal medicine.

State and Regional Veterinary Holistic Associations

Some of these organizations meet regularly and sponsor seminars on alternative treatments.

Florida Holistic Veterinary Medical Association
751 NE 168th Street
North Miami Beach, FL 33162-2427
Phone: 305-652-5372
Fax: 305-653-7244

Georgia Holistic Veterinary Medical Association
334 Knollwood Lane
Woodstock, GA 30188
Phone: 770-424-6303
E-mail: swynn@emory.edu

Great Lakes Holistic Veterinary Medical Association (mostly Illinois and Wisconsin)
9824 Durand Avenue
Sturtevant, WI 53177
Phone: 414-886-1100
Fax: 414-886-6460

Greater Washington Area Holistic Veterinary Association
6136 Brandon Avenue
Springfield, VA 22150
Phone: 703-503-8690

Rocky Mountain Holistic Veterinary Medical Association
311 S. Pennsylvania Street
Denver, CO 80209
Phone: 303-733-2728
Fax: 303-733-2858

Recommended Reading

Aromatherapy

Gattefosse, R. 1937. *Gattefosse's aromatherapy*. Essex, England: The C. W. Daniel Company.

Lawless, J. 1992. *The encyclopedia of essential oils*. Rockport, Massachusetts: Element, Inc.

Tisserand, R. 1977. *The art of aromatherapy*. Rochester, Vermont: Healing Arts Press.

Tisserand, R., and T. Balacs. 1995. *Essential oil safety: A guide for health professionals*. New York: Churchill Livingstone.

Ayurveda

Frawley, D. 1989. *Ayurvedic healing*. Salt Lake City, Utah: Passage Press.

Vasant, L. 1984. *Ayurveda: The science of self healing*. Santa Fe, New Mexico: Lotus Press.

Cancer Therapy

Boik, J. 1995. *Cancer and natural medicine: A textbook of basic science and clinical research*. Princeton, Minnesota: Oregon Medical Press.

Pelton, R., and L. Overholser. 1994. *Alternatives in cancer therapy*. New York: Simon and Schuster.

Complementary Medicine, General Reference

Fugh-Berman, A. 1996. *Alternative medicine: What works.* Tucson, Arizona: Odonian Press.

Lewith, G., J. Kenyon, and P. Lewis. 1996. *Complementary medicine: An integrated approach.* New York: Oxford University Press.

Spencer, J.W., and J.J. Jacobs. 1999. *Complementary/alternative medicine: An evidence based approach.* St. Louis, Missouri: Mosby.

Complementary Veterinary Medicine

Biddis, K.J. 1987. *Homeopathy in veterinary practice.* Essex, England: The C.W. Daniel Co., Ltd.

Coffman, H. 1996. *The dry dog food reference.* Nashua, New Hampshire: PigDog Press.

Day, C. 1984. *The homeopathic treatment of small animals: Principles and practice.* Essex, England: The C.W. Daniel Co., Ltd.

Fox, M. 1990. *The healing touch.* New York: Newmarket Press.

Janssens, L., and J. Still. 1995. *Acupuncture points and meridians in the dog.* Longmont, Colorado: IVAS.

Klide, A., and S. Kung. 1977. *Veterinary acupuncture.* Philadelphia: University of Pennsylvania Press.

Macleod, G. 1983. *Dogs: Homeopathic remedies.* Essex, England: The C.W. Daniel Co., Ltd.

Macleod, G. 1983. *A veterinary materia medical and clinical repertory, with a materia medical of the nosodes.* Essex, England: The C.W. Daniel Co., Ltd.

Macleod, G. 1990. *Cats: Homeopathic remedies.* Essex, England: The C.W. Daniel Co., Ltd.

Pitcairn, R., and S. Pitcairn. 1995. *Natural health for dogs and cats.* Emmaus, Pennsylvania: Rodale Press.

Schoen, A. 1994. *Veterinary acupuncture: Ancient art to modern medicine.* Indianapolis, Indiana: Mosby.

Schoen, A., and S. Wynn. 1997. *Complementary and alternative veterinary medicine: Principles and practice.* St. Louis, Missouri: Mosby.

Schwartz, C. 1996. *Four paws, five directions.* Berkeley, California: Celestial Arts Publishing.

Still, J. 1991. *Research in veterinary acupuncture.* Brussels, Belgium: Belgian Veterinary Acupuncture Society.

Strombeck, D. 1998. *Home prepared dog and cat diets*. Ames: Iowa State University Press.

Tellington-Jones, L. 1992. *The Tellington TTouch*. New York: Viking Penguin.

Xie, H. 1994. *Traditional Chinese veterinary medicine*. Beijing, China: Beijing Agricultural University Press.

Zidonis, N., and A. Snow. 1999. *The well-connected dog: A guide to canine acupressure*. Denver, Colorado: Tallgrass Publishers LLC.

Environmental Medicine

Carson, R. 1962. *Silent spring*. Boston: Houghton Mifflin Co.

Chivian, E., M. McCally, H. Hu, and A. Haines. 1993. *Critical condition: Human health and the environment*. Cambridge, Massachusetts: The MIT Press.

Rea, W.J. 1992. *Chemical sensitivity*. 4 Vols. Boca Raton, Florida: Lewis Publishers.

Herbal Medicine

Bissett, N. 1994. *Herbal drugs and phytopharmaceuticals: A handbook for practice on a scientific basis*. Boca Raton, Florida: CRC Press.

Blumenthal, M., and A. Goildberg, eds. 1998. *The German Commission E monographs*. Austin, Texas: American Botanical Council.

Bone, K. 1996. *Clinical applications of Ayurvedic and Chinese herbs: Monographs for the western herbal practitioner*. Warwick, Australia: Phytotherapy Press.

Cammarata, J. 1996. *A physician's guide to herbal wellness*. Chicago: Chicago Review Press.

De Smet, P.A.G., K. Keller, R. Hansel, and R.F. Chandler, eds. 1993. *Adverse effects of herbal drugs*. 3 Vols. New York: Springer-Verlag.

Fetrow, C.W., and J.R. Avib. 1999. *Professional's handbook of complementary and alternative medicines*. Springhouse, Pennsylvania: Springhouse.

Miller, L., and W. Murray. 1998. *Herbal medicinals: A clinician's guide*. New York: Pharmaceutical Products Press.

PDR for herbal medicines. 1998. Des Moines, Iowa: Medical Economics Company.

Pengelly, A. 1997. *The constituents of medicinal plants.* Merriwa, Australia: Sunflower Herbals. (U.S. distributor: Herbalist and Alchemist 800-611-8235, Broadway, NJ)

Schulz, V., R. Hansel, and V. Tyler. 1998. *Rational phytotherapy: A physician's guide to herbal medicine.* New York: Springer-Verlag.

Tyler, V. 1994. *Herbs of choice: The therapeutic use of phytomedicinals.* New York: Haworth Press.

Weiss, R. 1994. *Herbal medicine.* Beaconsfield, England: Beaconsfield Publishers Ltd.

Werbach, M., and M. Murray. 1994. *Botanical influences on illness: A sourcebook on clinical research.* Tarzana, California: Third Line Press, Inc.

Homeopathy

Bellavite, P. 1995. *Homeopathy: A frontier in medical science.* Experimental Studies and Theoretical Foundations. Berkeley, California: North Atlantic Books.

Bidwell, G. 1987. *How to use the repertory.* New Delhi, India: B. Jain Publishers.

Clarke, J.H. 1921. *A dictionary of practical materia medica.* 3 Vols. New Delhi, India: B. Jain Publishers.

Hahnemann, S. 1833. *Organon of medicine.* New Delhi, India: B. Jain Publishers.

Jayasuriya, A. 1993. *A complete course on clinical homeopathy.* New Delhi, India: B. Jain Publishers.

Morrison, R. 1993. *Desktop guide to keynotes and confirmatory symptoms.* Albany, California: Hahnemann Clinic Publishing.

Murphy, R. 1993. *Homeopathic medical repertory.* Pagosa Springs, Colorado: Hahnemann Academy of North America.

Sankaran, R. 1991. *The spirit of homeopathy.* Bombay, India: Homeopathic Medical Publishers.

Vithoulkas, G. 1980. *The science of homeopathy.* New York: Grove Press, Inc.

Naturopathy

Murray, M., and J. Pizzorno. 1997. *Encyclopedia of natural medicine.* Rocklin, California: Prima Publishing.

Nutrition

Lopez, D.A., R.M. Williams, and M. Miehlke. 1994. *Enzymes: The fountain of life*. Charleston, North Carolina: The Neville Press, Inc.

Werbach, M. 1987. *Nutritional influences on illness: A sourcebook of clinical research*. Tarzana, California: Third Line Press, Inc.

Werbach, M. 1997. *Foundations of nutritional medicine*. Tarzana, California: Third Line Press, Inc.

Traditional Chinese Medicine

Bensky, D., and R. Barolet. 1993. *Chinese herbal medicine: Formulas and strategies*. Seattle, Washington: Eastland Press, Inc.

Bensky, D., and A. Gamble. 1993. *Chinese herbal medicine: Materia medica*. Seattle, Washington: Eastland Press, Inc.

Fratkin, J. 1986. *Chinese herbal patent formulas: A practical guide*. Boulder, Colorado: SHYA Publications.

Huang, K.C. 1998. *The pharmacology of Chinese herbs*. Boca Raton, Florida: CRC Press.

Kaptchuk, T. 1983. *The web that has no weaver: Understanding Chinese medicine*. New York: Congdon and Weed.

Maciocia, G. 1989. *The foundations of Chinese medicine*. New York: Churchill Livingstone.

Maciocia, G. 1994. *The practice of Chinese medicine*. New York: Churchill Livingstone.

Reid, D.P. 1986. *Chinese herbal medicine*. Boston: Shambhala Publications Inc.

Websites

Acupuncture
Acupuncture.Com
    http://www.Acupuncture.com
Australian Medical Acupuncture Society
    http://www.ozacupuncture.com
The Medical Acupuncture Page
    http://www.med.auth.gr/~karanik/english/main.htm

Alternative Medicine
Alternative Health News Online
    http://www.altmedicine.com/
The Alternative Medicine Homepage
    http://www.pitt.edu/~cbw/altm.html
Office of Alternative Medicine
    http://altmed.od.nih.gov/nccam

Alternative Veterinary Medicine
Academy of Veterinary Homeopathy
    http://www.acadvethom.org
AltVetMed—general information, introductory material
    http://www.altvetmed.com
American Veterinary Chiropractic Association
    http://www.healthworld.com/pan/pa/vet/avca/
International Veterinary Acupuncture Society
    http://www.ivas.org

The Veterinary Acupuncture Page—veterinary acupuncture—clinical and scientific

> http://www.med.auth.gr/~karanik/english/veter.htm

Chiropractic

Chiro-Web

> http://pages.prodigy.com/CT/doc/doc.html

Electrical Hypersensitivity

Electrosensitivity

> http://www.feb.se/

Herbs

American Botanical Council

> www.herbalgram.org/

Health World Online Herbal Materia Medica

> http://www.healthy.net/clinic/therapy/herbal/herbic/herbs/index.html

Herb Research Foundation

> http://www.herbs.org/

Michael Moore's SW School of Botanical Medicine

> http://chili.rt66.com/hrbmoore/HOMEPAGE/HomePage.html

Phytochemical and Ethnobotanical Database

> http://www.ars-grin.gov/~ngrlsb

Chinese Herbs

Rocky Mountain Herbal Institute

> http://www.rmhiherbal.org/

Traditional Chinese Medicine

> http://www.tcm.org.uk/

Homeopathy

Caduceus Institute of Classical Homeopathy

> http://www.homeopathyhome.com

Homeopathy Online (online journal of homeopathy)

> http://www.lyghtforce.com/HomeopathyOnline/

National Center for Homeopathy

> http://www.healthy.net/associations/pa/Homeopathic/Natcenhom/

Nutraceuticals

FDA Adverse Reporting Page for Nutritional Supplements

> http://vm.cfsan.fda.gov/~dms/aems.html

NIH Office of Dietary Supplements—IBIDS Database
http://odp.od.nih.gov/ods/databases/ibids.html

Oriental Medicine

Journal of Chinese Medicine
http://www.pavilion.co.uk/jcm/welcome.html

Traditional/Ethnobotanical Medicine

Institute for Traditional Medicine
http://www.itmonline.org

Periodicals

The periodicals in this section are primarily of general interest; specialty journals in Chinese medicine, homeopathy, massage, acupuncture, herbs, phytopharmacognosy, and many other areas are available to more advanced practitioners.

Alternative and Complementary Therapies
Mary Ann Liebert, Inc., Publishers
2 Madison Avenue
Larchmont, NY 10538
Phone: 914-834-3100
Fax: 914-834-3771

Alternative Medicine Review
Thorne Research, Inc.
P.O. Box 3200
Sandpoint, ID 83864
Phone: 208-263-1337
Fax: 208-265-2488

Alternative Therapies in Health and Medicine
101 Columbia
Aliso Viejo, CA 92656
Phone: 800-899-1712

Clinical Pearls News
IT Services
3301 Alta Arden #3
Sacramento, CA 95825
Phone: 800-422-9887

FACT: Focus on Alternative and Complementary Therapies
Verlag PERFUSION GmbH
Regensburgerstr 44-46
90478 Nurnberg
Germany

Health Inform: Essential Information on Alternative Health Care
InfoLink
P.O. Box 306
31 Albany Post Road
Montrose, NY 10548
Phone: 914-736-1565
Fax: 914-736-3806

Herbalgram
American Botanical Council
P.O. Box 201660
Austin, TX 78720
Phone: 512-331-8868

International Journal of Integrative Medicine
Impakt Communications, Inc.
P.O. Box 12496
Green Bay, WI 54307-2496
Phone: 414-499-2995
Fax: 414-499-3441

Journal of Alternative and Complementary Medicine
Mary Ann Liebert, Inc., Publishers
2 Madison Avenue
Larchmont, NY 10538
Phone: 914-834-3100
Fax: 914-834-3771

Journal of the American Holistic Veterinary Medical Association
2214 Old Emmorton Road
Bel Air, MD 21015
Phone: 410-569-0795
E-mail: AHVMA@compuserve.com

Medical Herbalism: A Clinical Newsletter for the Herbal Practitioner
Bergner Communications
P.O. Box 33080
Portland, OR 97233
Phone: 800-231-9290

Modern Phytotherapist
Professional Health Products LTD
LPN Sales
P.O. Box 2046
Warrendale, PA 15086-2046
E-mail: www.mediherb.com.au

Practical Reviews of Complementary and Alternative Medicine
Educational Reviews, LLC
6801 Cahaba Valley Road
Birmingham, AL 35242-9988
Phone: 800-633-4743; 205-991-5188
Fax: 205-995-1926
E-mail: www.edreview.com

Quarterly Review of Natural Medicine
NPRC
600 First Avenue
Suite 205
Seattle, WA 98104
Phone: 206-623-2520

Suppliers

Books and Information

Homeopathic Educational Services
2124 Kittredge Street
Berkeley, CA 94704
Phone: 800-359-9051

Redwing Book Company
44 Linden Street
Brookline, MA 02146
Phone: 617-738-4664
> Large and varied selection, but concentrates on traditional Chinese medicine.

Veterinary Supplies

Advanced Biological Concepts
301 Main Street
P.O. Box 27
Osco, IL 61274
Phone: 800-373-5971
Canada: 800-779-3959
Fax: 309-522-5570
> Nutritional and herbal products.

Animals' Apawthecary
P.O. Box 212
Conner, MT 59827
Phone: 406-821-4090
　Herbs.

Dr. Goodpet
P.O. Box 4489
Inglewood, CA 90309
Phone: 800-222-0032
　Combination homeopathics and nutritional supplements.

Fleabusters/Rx for Fleas
2262 NW Parkway, Suite 1
Marietta, GA 30067
Phone: 404-956-0555
　Sodium polyborate powder.

Hilton Herbs, Ltd.
Downclose Farm
North Perott, Crewkerne
Somerset TA18 7SH
England
American distributor (Echo Publishing): 505-989-7280
　Western herbal combinations for dogs and horses.

Natural Animal, Inc.
P.O. Box 1177
St. Augustine, FL 32085
Phone: 800-274-7387
　Natural flea control products, Ester-C.

Natural Animal Nutrition
Bel Air, MD
Phone: 800-548-2899
　Nutritional supplements.

Nutramax
8304 Harford Road
Baltimore, MD 21234
Phone: 800-925-5187
   Nutraceuticals.

Orthomolecular Specialties
P.O. Box 32232
San Jose, CA 95152-2232
Phone: 408-227-9334
   Nutritional supplements.

PetSage
4313 Wheeler Avenue
Alexandria, VA 22304
Phone: 800-PET-HLTH
   Retail distributor for many herbs, nutraceuticals, etc.

Rx Vitamins for Pets
200 Myrtle Boulevard
Larchmont, NY 10538
Phone: 800-792-2222; 914-834-1804
Website: www.rxvitamins.com

Springtime Feed Company
10942-J Beaver Dam Road
P.O. Box 1227
Cockeysville, MD 21030
Phone: 800-521-3212
   Nutritional/herb mixed supplements.

Vetri-Science Laboratories
20 New England Drive-C 1504
Essex Junction, VT 05453-1504
Phone: 800-882-9993
   Nutritional supplements.

Wysong
1880 North Eastman Road
Midland, MI 48640
Phone: 800-748-0188
  Foods, some herbal therapeutics.

Natural Products, Miscellaneous

Advanced Medical Nutrition, Inc. (AMNI)
2247 National Avenue
P.O. Box 5012
Hayward, CA 94540-5012
Phone: 800-654-4432

Allergy Research Group
400 Preda Street
San Leandro, CA 94577-0489
Phone: 510-487-8526

Douglas Laboratories
600 Boyce Road
Pittsburgh, PA 15205
Phone: 800-245-4440
Fax: 412-494-0155
  Large selection of nutritional supplements, some herbs.

ICN Pharmaceuticals
3300 Hyland Avenue
Costa Mesa, CA 92626
Phone: 800-533-1033

Metagenics
971 Calle Negocio
San Clemente, CA 92672
Phone: 800-692-9400

Nubiologics, Inc.
2470 Wisconsin Avenue
Downers Grove, IL 60515
Phone: 800-332-3130
  Nutrition/glandular supplements.

Professional Health Products LTD
LPN Sales
P.O. Box 2046
Warrendale, PA 15086-2046

Pure Encapsulations
490 Boston Post Road
Sudbury, MA 01776
Phone: 800-753-2277

Thorne Research
25820 Highway 2 West
P.O. Box 25
Dover, ID 83825
Phone: 800-228-1966
208-263-1337
Fax: 208-265-2488
E-mail: www.thorne.com

Torrance Co.
800 Lenox Avenue
Partage, MI 49002
Phone: 800-327-0722
    Injectable vitamins.

Tyler Encapsulations
2204-8 N.W. Birdsdale
Gresham, OR 97030
Phone: 800-869-9705

Herbs

Ayush Herbs, Inc.
2115 112th NE
Bellevue, WA 98006
Phone: 425-637-1400
Fax: 425-451-2670
E-mail: ayurveda@ayush.com
    Ayurvedic herbs.

Brion Corporation
9200 Jeronimo Road
Irvine, CA 92718
Phone: 800-333-4372
Chinese herbs, Sun Ten formulas.

East Coast Herbs Distributor
2525 South Mount Juliet Road
Mt. Juliet, TN 37122
Phone: 800-283-5191
Distributor for Brion (Chinese) herbs.

Golden Flower Chinese Herbs
P.O. Box 781
Placitas, NM 87043
Phone: 800-729-8509
Chinese herbs.

Health Concerns
8001 Capwell Drive
Oakland, CA 94621
Phone: 800-233-9355
Chinese herbal combinations.

Herb Pharm
P.O. Box 116
Williams, OR 97544
Phone: 800-348-4372
Fax: 541-846-6112
Single herbs in tincture, Western with some Chinese and Ayurvedic.

Institute of Traditional Medicine
2017 SE Hawthorne
Portland, OR 97214
Phone: 503-233-4907
Seven Forest Chinese herbal formulas, reference materials.

K'an Herb Company
6001 Butler Lane
Scotts Valley, CA 95066
Phone: 831-438-9450
    Chinese herbal combinations.

MayWay Trading Company
1338 Cypress Street
Oakland, CA 94607
Phone: 510-208-3113
    Chinese patent herbs, single herbs.

Nature's Way and Murdock` Pharmaceuticals, Inc.
1400 Mountain Springs Park
Springville, UT 84663
Phone: 800-962-8873
    Western herbs.

Nuherbs Co.
3820 Penniman Avenue
Oakland, CA 94519
Phone: 800-233-4307
    Chinese patent herbs.

NutriWest–China West
P.O. Box 950
Douglas, WY 82633
Phone: 800-443-3333

Zand Herbal Formulas
P.O. Box 5312
Santa Monica, CA 90409
Phone: 800-800-0405
    Chinese herbs, tinctures.

Index

Note: f. indicates figure; t. indicates table.